Praise for *Jiffy Body*

Succinct explanations and extensive variations on exercise routines suited to a wide range of abilities, this is an inviting tool for achieving better health.
—*Publishers Weekly* review in the Best the Books and Authors section

The Jiffy Body system is logical and simple to implement. This non-workout is easy to follow and super effective. What a great advantage to learn simple tricks and techniques to get your body to feel and function better.

—Patrick Mckeown, author of the bestselling
The Oxygen Advantage

The Jiffy Body book has been a help to me in numerous ways. I suffer from chronic low back pain and left hip pain. By reading this book and following the instructions that Bart discusses I have experienced relief in my problem areas. My goal is to improve further and prevent other painful issues in other joints. The book is concise, easy to read and the pictures are excellent. I highly recommend *Jiffy Body* for those people with or without pain.

— Paul Bregman MD Denver, CO

Being a senior in my 70's, to my delight, the Jiffy Body System deleted the low back¬pain I have suffered with for at least 35 years. The squeaking hip joint problem and plantar fasciitis are also gone! I do the exercises 1 or 2 times a day. Very relaxing with my dog on the floor! A renewed body and no more pain meds! Extremely happy!

—Agneta, Amazon reviewer

My balance has improved, the aches and pains are no longer an issue, and my posture is much better. There is no doubt in my mind that the Jiffy Body tune up can improve the performance of every active individual regardless of age due to the resulting enhanced flexibility and balance. Now that I have read *Jiffy Body* it is my constant companion for continued performance improvement many years ahead.　　　　　　　　—Dynamo, Amazon reviewer

Jiffy Body gives you a simple, quick plan to develop and maintain natural movement from head to toe. I encourage you to try it (and enjoy it) and feel the changes in your body.
　　　　　　　　　　　　—Steven Sashen, CEO Xero Shoes

Being a Health Coach and former Massage Therapist, I realize the importance of musculoskeletal health. Bart's book, *Jiffy Body,* brings a simple approach to daily routines that will relieve discomforts and improve performance (simple daily tasks or more strenuous movements). This is a go-to solution for anyone living in pain!
　　　　—Connie Pshigoda, author of *The Wise Woman's Almanac*

I was introduced to these practices when Bart was doing his apprenticeship and they deliver results as promised! I have used the techniques intermittently over the years "as needed." In the past year or so I have incorporated them into my daily routines in order to avoid pain and also to alleviate pain as it occurs. The practices are simple and yet powerfully effective. I recommend this book to anyone that deals with or wants to avoid joint pain.
　　　　　　　　　　　　　　　　　　— Lisa Klein

A few months ago I started feeling aches and pains throughout my body. After reading and following Bart's instructions in his book, *Jiffy Body,* I have felt those pains less and less over time. I am very pleased with what he teaches and am very much looking forward to a pain free life. I highly recommend this book to anyone who wants the same.
　　　　　　　　　　　　　　　　　—Robin Heykoop

Bart at Jiffy Body really knows his stuff. His book is great because it clearly walks you through the why's and how's of taking care of your body for the rest of your life. I love Bart's program! It is accessible, affordable and effective!

—Susan Bickel

The book outlines a very simple approach to help realign muscle groups to aid with body posture and pain relief. I found the descriptions, explanations and photos very helpful and noticed quick results using the author's techniques! I can highly recommend this book!

—Katherine Montgomery, Amazon reviewer

I train with weights daily and have had my own stretching/rolling routine for years gathered from multiple online sources. I've been able to stave off injury with my routine but Bart's system and the way he explains the muscles in *Jiffy Body* has greatly improved my workouts and mobility in general. The book is a must for sedentary job-goers but also extremely helpful for fitness.

— Daniel Battersby

I worked with Bart one on one in the past with tremendous success. I would start feeling better and needed to see Bart less. After a while I had trouble trying to remember the tools Bart had shown me. Over time I would go back to Bart for a refresher. This book is so easy to read and follow as if Bart is in the room instructing me all over again. Plus, there's techniques I haven't worked with yet. I'm an electrician and handyman. I'm pretty hard on my body I found the Jiffy Body system really keeps my body in the shape my job demands. Thank you Bart.

— Jacob Medrano

Absolutely the best $20 I've ever spent. *Jiffy Body* is an easy read and it delivers great results. I've made the exercises and stretches part of my daily routine and I haven't felt this good in years. The Jiffy Body book makes it all make sense.

—Steve Antonczyk, General Manager, Colorado Home Fitness

JIFFY

BODY™

The 10-Minute System to Avoid Joint and Muscle Pain

BART POTTER

JIFFY BODY™:
The 10-Minute System to Avoid Joint and Muscle Pain
by Bart Potter

Always consult your physician or healthcare professional before beginning any exercise program. This general information is not intended to diagnose any medical condition or to replace your healthcare professional. Consult with your healthcare professional to design an appropriate exercise and/or physical therapy prescription. If you experience any numbness, tingling, pain or difficulty with these exercises, stop and consult your healthcare professional.

Published by Blue River Publishing
Littleton, CO

ISBN: 978-1-7339843-0-0
LCCN: 2019907726

Cover and Interior Design by Nick Zelinger, NZ Graphics.com
Photography by Denise Stein
Editing by Jennifer Jas
Modeling by Linda Futrell and Bart Potter
Anatomy Illustrations by Ankita and Robin Mishra
Cartoons by Greg Houston

HEA018000 HEALTH & FITNESS / Physical Impairments
HEA009000 HEALTH & FITNESS / Healing
HEA032000 HEALTH & FITNESS / Alternative Therapies

First Edition

Printed in the United States of America

How to Use This Book

First, learn the principles of this system in Parts One, Two and Three before practicing in Part Four. You may be tempted to fast-forward straight to a section of your body that you want to work on.

Keep in mind that there isn't a single body part that works independently of the others. For example, if you have an ankle problem, you could feel the effect all the way into your hips or lower back (and vice versa). For this reason, it can be helpful to look away from a challenged body part to improve. Plus, your whole body benefits by practicing the entire system!

As you read Part Three, do not practice all of the positions demonstrated in that section. There are numerous extra positions included with varying degrees of difficulty. That way when you begin practice (in Part Four), you will have options that work best for your body.

The 10-minute system is demonstrated in Part Four. It consists of up to 17 positions. You can run through all of them in 10 minutes (after you have run through the system several times).

Here's the catch. Once you learn the system, you will need to practice the positions (up to 10 minutes per day is all). But if you are willing to do that, then Jiffy Body will work for you!

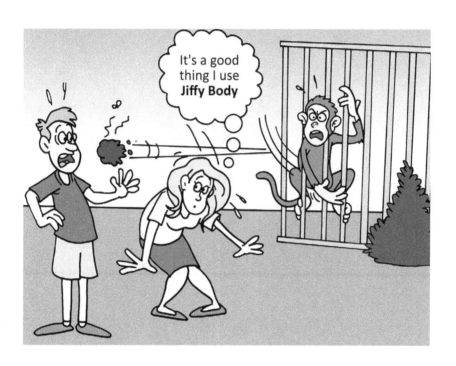

CONTENTS

PART ONE

OUR BODY BRIDGE AND THE PAIN ALARM

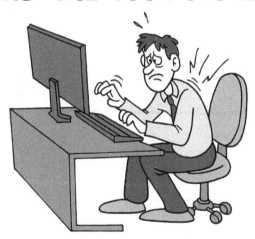

Muscle Imbalance—Causing Aches, Pains and Injuries

When gravity tries to drag and pull us down all day, what is it that keeps our bones from falling to the ground like a sack of dirt?

Answer: Our heroic muscles! They defeat gravity and maintain an upright structure (bones and joints)!

They also balance our structure, similar to the way steel cables support, balance and distribute the weight of a suspension bridge. However, your "body bridge" isn't stuck in one spot. You can take it for a walk, go dancing or play on the floor, while your muscles keep your bones and joints in balance. That's truly amazing. We are all walking miracles!

Problems happen when your "muscle cable" tension is imbalanced. That pulls your body bridge off-center, causing structural problems (in particular, joint injuries). It also causes muscle symptoms like aches, pains, stiffness and restricted blood flow.

Here's a simple example. Sitting in cars, couches and chairs is a major culprit for causing muscle imbalance between the upper front muscles and upper back muscles.

Upper Front Muscles

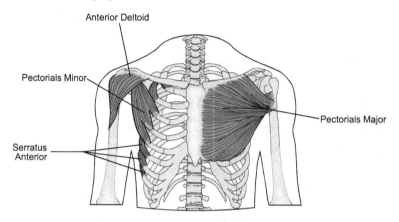

Upper Back Muscles

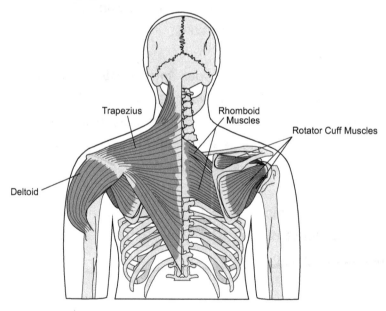

Because many of these muscles overlap, they are shown in both pictures using the right and left sides of the body. That way you can see all of them at once.

While sitting most people tend to hunch over their computers, steering wheels and even slouch in their couches. **As a result, the upper front muscles shorten, and the upper back muscle cables overstretch.**

If you sit 40+ hours a week like this, your "muscle cables" are off-balance **the entire time**. Then when you get up and move, you can take this imbalance with you. "Practicing" like this for weeks and even years can create aches, pains and injuries for the shoulders, neck and upper back. It can even restrict blood flow and cause headaches.

Your body actually warns you with these symptoms to discourage you from using misaligned, injury-prone parts. **By identifying common muscle imbalances and taking simple steps to correct them, your joints and muscles will feel and perform better.**

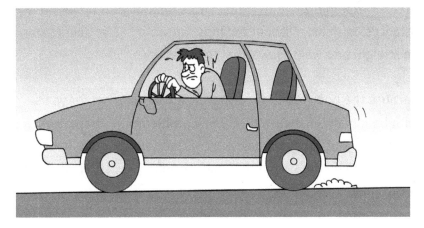

Sitting in a chair and car: Notice that the shoulders, neck and head are too far forward and off-center! Over time this lopsided position can create structural problems, in particular for the joints in the neck and shoulders.

High-Performance Living Machinery

Let's first acknowledge that we are all lucky owners of the most impressive machinery on the planet. Even if you just look at the location of your joints, you'll notice an elegant symmetry from the top to the bottom. Your shoulders and hips are both ball-and-socket joints. That's why you can use them both with impressive variety.

The elbows look and function similarly to the knees (both hinge joints). The smaller joints in our hands look and function similarly to the smaller joints in our feet. They all provide us the ability for precision movement and expression.

Let's put it this way: If your joints were an 80s band, they would definitely be Bon Jovi. That's right, they are rock stars!

Take for example your hip joints. The weight of your upper body balances on them. Without the hips, we wouldn't be able to stand up straight and walk. How's that for a benefit!

Because the body is designed so well, it can run great for years with little maintenance and very few problems. In comparison, if you drove your car every day for years without tuneups, it would break down on the side of the road (hopefully my sister will hear about this).

Sometimes it can be hard to truly appreciate your joints and body mechanics until you have trouble with one or more of your parts.

My Experience with Chronic Pain

When I was growing up, I used my body relentlessly without a problem and just expected it to work great. I was always moving: playing with our huge family dogs, neighborhood kids, and pretending I was Huckleberry Finn and exploring the river we lived next to. Being physically active and playing outdoors were the norm back then. After all, there weren't any smartphones.

I also spent countless hours chasing around tennis balls on asphalt courts. Back then there was a famous tennis player named Bjorn Borg. He was so amazing he actually made tennis a popular sport and I hoped to one day play professionally like him.

Playing that much tennis over a 12-year stretch is kind of like painting your house with a paintbrush using one arm. At first, it's no problem. But as you continue to paint your house, then your neighbor's and your mom's house, eventually your arm and shoulder are screaming.

As I logged countless hours of practice, by high school my body protested with aches, pains, stiffness and swelling. Those warnings were useful. If there was no pain alarm, we would just keep using and further damaging our dysfunctional parts.

In response, I sought out experts in sports medicine and physical therapy. As captain of both my high school and college tennis teams, I implemented warm-up, stretching and training techniques as part of our daily practice. Still, I experienced symptoms and dysfunction from swinging a racket with maximum velocity and sprinting on asphalt. As a result, my body progressively turned up the pain and inflammation alarm.

Trying to Ignore Pain

Many of my clients have had a similar experience. At first, they felt nagging symptoms which they could ignore. However, they didn't fix the cause of the problem and so their symptoms intensified. Eventually, it was like their bodies were yelling at them.

In high school and college, I was determined to keep playing regardless of the warning signs. Tennis is a lopsided sport like golf where you use muscles more consistently on one side of the body. That creates muscle imbalance and pulls the structure (bones and joints) off-center. I didn't understand how to counter this effect, despite having consulted experts in muscles, bones and body rehabilitation.

If my body could have talked to me, it would have said something like, "Hey dummy, quit playing tennis or I'm going to completely cut you off from the use of your shoulder." By my junior year in college, my shoulder was screaming at me. I couldn't swing a racket for five minutes without pain.

So I finally listened and gave up tennis and also the dream of one day playing professionally. It would have been so easy to avoid this outcome with the knowledge and techniques I eventually learned from a master human body mechanic!

Common Causes of Muscle Imbalance

As mentioned earlier, sitting can create muscle imbalance. A large majority of us (myself included) count sitting as one of our top activities. You may notice after a sitting session that it's harder to stand up straight and walk. That's because your body readjusts your "muscle cable" tension to support sitting, not standing and movement.

When it comes to muscle imbalance, your body produces what you practice most consistently.

Following are examples of the most common muscle imbalances caused by sitting, **especially if nothing is done to counteract them.**

- Most people tend to roll back on their butt, instead of forward onto the pelvis. As they roll back, the arch flattens in the lower spine. A "flattened" arch causes a disappearing butt while standing and walking. It also hinders movement and can spur back pain and dysfunction. Plus, it decreases your chances of getting cast in a music video.

- The knees are bent, which tightens the hamstrings (a group of three muscles on the upper back part of the legs). When hamstrings are excessively tight, they exert downward pressure on the pelvis, which can once again "flatten" the arch in the lower spine and cause pain.

- Hip joints are flexed (pulled toward the upper body). Hip flexion is a natural movement. However, it becomes a problem for hip longevity and function when the hip joints are stuck in this position for an excessive amount of time.

- Hip flexor muscles enable your legs to move up toward your body. These muscles tighten while you sit. Tight hip flexors disrupt movement and are notorious for causing back pain.

Wow, that's a lot of muscle imbalances and potential joint and pain problems caused by sitting!

If you don't counteract them, these seated muscle patterns can become locked in and follow you everywhere. You could be in a yoga class, dancing or on the golf course and suddenly your back seizes up. Then you might think, "I shouldn't do this activity anymore because my back can't handle it."

In fact, we all create our own unique set of muscle imbalances by the most consistent activities we participate in. Over years of time, these imbalances can cause unnecessary pain, damage joints and limit our ability to have fun using our amazing living machinery.

The more hours you spend on repetitive activities (like sitting), the more specific actions you need to take to counteract that activity (to avoid muscle imbalance, pain and injury). For this reason, Part Four includes simple steps to counteract the muscle imbalances and joint constriction caused by sitting.

Following are a few more examples of common muscle imbalances which can also result in restricted joint function. Page numbers are included to reference simple tactics in the book for counteracting muscle imbalance and creating better joint function.

Walking for Exercise: Muscle Imbalance and Joint Dysfunction
If you walk a lot for exercise and don't stretch your hamstrings and calves, they can get progressively tighter. This disrupts how your feet impact the ground. The hamstring tightness also pulls down on the back side of your pelvis. This can cause the lower arch in your spine to flatten. These muscle imbalances can cause joint problems in the feet, ankles, knees, hips and lower spine.

Calf and hamstring stretches are highlighted on pages 45-61.

Hips and Shoulders: Muscle Imbalance and Joint Dysfunction
Our hip and shoulder joints are healthier and last longer when we use them with effective range of motion. The problem is that most of us spend the bulk of our days seated on couches, in cars and in front of computers (using limited joint range of motion).

Even 100 years ago people didn't have that luxury. They had to work and use their bodies for a wide range of chores and activities. That forced their muscles and joints to provide more complete and effective joint range of motion.

Because of a modern, more sedentary lifestyle, we don't have to do nearly as much manual labor. That limits the use of our joints and supporting muscles. **Not using joint range of motion often leads to losing joint range of motion and decreasing muscle balance.** This can cause three main joint problems:

- Unpleasant symptoms like aches, pains, stiffness and swelling.

- Restricted function making it harder to use joints.

- Instability which increases injury potential, loss of coordination and more rapid joint degradation.

For example, a client came to me with a self-described "frozen shoulder." She hadn't sustained any single injury. Instead, she noticed losing normal range of motion in her right shoulder over time. Everyday tasks like pulling a glass out of a cabinet had become painful. She couldn't sleep on her right side as well because that shoulder was so uncomfortable.

She regained full function and eliminated painful symptoms by 1) restoring upper body muscle balance and 2) practicing shoulder range of motion exercises.

Restoring upper body muscle balance and shoulder range of motion practice positions are highlighted on pages 84-100.

Modern Technology: Muscle Imbalance and Joint Dysfunction
Some kids and adults play video games or use their phones endlessly, which sometimes turns them into zombies.

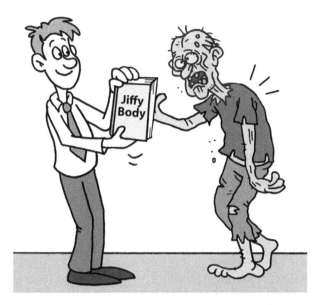

So simple it works for everyone, even a zombie.

Hunching over phones and repetitively using wrists and fingers create excessive muscle tightness in the upper body, forearms and hands. These muscles constrict nerve pathways that supply the shoulders, elbows, wrists and hands with power. That leads to aches, pains and swelling in these parts.

A specific practice plan for counteracting shoulder and wrist dysfunction is located on pages 84-101.

Constricted Toe Joints: Muscle Imbalance and Joint Dysfunction
Our feet contain lots of small joints (similar to our hands). **They benefit by being allowed to express normal range of motion (as with all of our other joints).** Wearing a straitjacket would cause shoulder pain and injury over time by constricting joint range of motion.

Similarly, most modern shoes restrict toe joint range of motion. They often squeeze the toes together in the front of the shoe. This is more prevalent with high heel women's shoes. However, there are even men's shoes that have a constricted toe box. This increases the likelihood of dysfunction, pain and injury over time.

If you crawled around on the floor, you would notice less balance when your fingers are not allowed to spread out. It's the same principle for your toes. The body is less stable when the toes (and supporting muscles) are prevented from spreading out with every step.

Elevated Heel: Muscle Imbalance and Joint Dysfunction
An elevated heel in most shoes pitches the body's center of gravity too far forward. Even men's shoes can have a heel higher than the toes. This pushes your "body bridge" off-center. The calves tighten, and more pressure is placed on smaller joints in the front of the foot.

Perhaps you already have foot concerns? If so, take a look at your shoes. The problems compound as the heel gets higher and the toes are more crammed together (which usually happens with fancier shoes).

This imbalance often results in aches, pains, restricted blood flow and swelling in the feet and ankles. It increases the chances of nerve impingement, plantar fasciitis, coordination problems and injury.

Keep in mind that overall body balance starts with your feet. When they are misaligned with improper footwear, that can create problems higher up the ladder (ankles, knees, hips, pelvis and lower back).

By wearing shoes without an elevated heel or a constricted toe box, you give your feet a break. If you do plan to change your type of shoes, at first wear the new ones minimally to let the muscles in your feet make a gradual adjustment.

My Own Assortment of Muscle Imbalances

In high school and college, I developed my own impressive array of muscle imbalances which led to joint dysfunction, pain and injury. As mentioned, tennis was a major cause because it is a "lopsided" sport.

My hamstrings were also excessively tight. That caused a flattened arch in the lower back, and eventually lower back pain. My upper body was off-balance from spending tons of hours hunched over studying at my desk (not to mention I was a natural sloucher).

Over time, this created tight upper front muscles and overstretched upper back muscles. As a result, the shoulder joints were pulled forward and off-center, which created joint instability and restricted range of motion. The right shoulder was also at least two inches lower than the left shoulder. Wow what a mess!

But wait, there's more!

After college, I moved to Colorado where I mountain biked, skied and hiked. All of my muscle imbalances came along with me! It was like trying to drive a car with the wheels out of alignment. After one very memorable ski accident, suddenly my right shoulder began to hurt every day. I came up with a solution that many people use when a body part consistently hurts. I simply used the right shoulder and supporting muscles less to try not to irritate them. This was not a successful tactic!

When you stop using muscles because of pain they shrink in size. For this reason, the muscles in my right shoulder, arm and hand were slowly disappearing. Eventually, these muscles contained half as much mass as the same muscles on the opposite side. My shoulder became so painful that I learned to write left-handed. Just playing guitar for 10 minutes was enough to cause shoulder pain for the rest of the day. So, I quit playing guitar and left the band I was in, as well.

I was in my 20s but sure didn't feel that way. Anyone who has had chronic pain will tell you it affects everything: how you walk, think and move. Perhaps you or a loved one have had a similar experience of making appointments with expert after expert without a solution. In my case, some of the experts even discounted the symptoms. Some doctors prescribed pills for the pain, but they didn't prescribe a plan to fix the cause of the problem.

I tried a wide range of Eastern and Western medicine. A chronic pain specialist stuck needles deep into my upper back muscles to release trigger points and hopefully decrease pain (since I had pain in my upper back as well). A sports medicine doctor who seemed perplexed on how to help me, said, "You know, some people just experience pain more easily than others."

I remember a doctor at Johns Hopkins Hospital on the East Coast telling me the muscles on my right side had atrophied so much they might not return to normal size.

I was fortunate to receive help from Florence Kendall, a well-known physical therapist, teacher and author. I met her through another physical therapist who thought I was an interesting and challenging case. Florence was retired but graciously agreed to help me for free.

Thanks to Florence, I was able to somewhat improve. Nevertheless, my shoulder, lower and upper back were still painful and dysfunctional. I was operating at around 10 percent of what I used to be able to do physically. I remember Florence telling me that my shoulder might not improve to the point that I could drive a car with a stick shift. That was a bummer because I wanted my next car to be a stick shift.

When you hear from numerous experts that there may not be a solution, you get to the point where you believe them. At this point, I lost hope and stopped seeking out help.

Meet the Ultimate Human Body Mechanic

Fortunately, both the experts and I turned out to be wrong. Also, I got extremely lucky. My parents had moved to Trinidad, a one-stoplight town in southern Colorado. To me, Trinidad looked like Colorado's version of that old hit TV show *Northern Exposure.* My mother (aka the happy wanderer), who talks to everyone, met a "fitness trainer" at the local gym on Main Street. She said he seemed really knowledgeable and confident he could help me.

Having already consulted so many people with advanced degrees and education, you can imagine I was super skeptical. It was hard to imagine that I would find a solution at a small-town gym. But pain is a powerful motivator. When you've had it long enough, you'll try just about anything to get better. You'll eventually quit a great job at a software company in Seattle and move to a tiny town in southern Colorado to improve.

When I first met Sean McCarver, I thought he looked like a pro wrestler or the head of a motorcycle gang. In reality, Sean was actually a big nerd when it came to the human body. His idea of a fun night was staying home and studying his worn-out anatomy and physiology textbooks. Sean had played in the NFL, fought professionally and excelled in power-lifting competitions. Throughout his career, his clients ranged from grandparents, parents and kids to college and professional athletes.

During his sports career, he had broken multiple bones, torn plenty of connective tissue and fractured his spine. He learned rehabilitation firsthand by fixing up his own broken body. At one point he had major back surgery and was confined to a wheelchair.

Since Sean admired cars and motorcycles, it made sense that he thought of our body parts as living machinery. He also problem-solved the body similar to the way a software developer writes code: patiently tweaking his approach to get the desired outcome. "Never use your education as a limitation," he often said.

A large number of Sean's clients were people who had tried a variety of Eastern and Western medicine first to fix pain and injuries. These were Sean's favorite clients. Because he had lived it, he had compassion for what they were going through.

Sean did not use expensive technology to analyze and treat patients with muscle and joint problems. However, he studied for thousands of hours and practiced his craft for over 30 years. Therefore, he developed a unique and effective approach to help clients tune up their living machinery.

Because of his unique insights, the solution to my joint and muscle pain ended up being so ridiculously simple. Within 30 minutes of our first meeting, I could tell right away that Sean knew exactly what to do. He implemented a two-part plan to get me back on track: 1) Identify muscle imbalance and 2) restore muscle balance to the affected body parts.

Sean's clients routinely achieved better body function and eliminated aches and pains by learning how to implement this two-part plan. He helped me get back to 100 percent and return to competitive tennis, hiking, skiing, surfing and playing guitar in a local folk band.

You can benefit from Sean's techniques as well. You'll learn to analyze and gain valuable information about your body mechanics. Then take simple actions to tune up your parts, improve function and create more stable, long-lasting joints.

I became so impressed with the results Sean achieved with his clients, that I apprenticed with him. I then used his approach to help my own clients with pain, dysfunction and fitness. *Jiffy Body* is based on more than 20 years of practice and refining Sean's ideas and creating great results for my clients. Sean has sadly passed away, but he would be thrilled to know that his ideas are alive and available to help you.

PART TWO

WHY JIFFY BODY WORKS FOR YOU

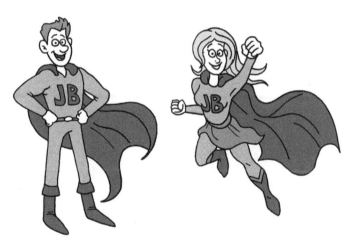

Think of this system as your body's own 28-point inspection—a systematic way to target living mechanical parts and take positive actions to benefit them by focusing on three key areas:

1. Restoring and Maintaining Muscle Balance

2. Restoring and Maintaining Effective Joint Range of Motion

3. Identifying and Improving Weak Points, and Preventing Injuries

The benefits of focusing on these three areas include:

1. Create better blood flow to your body parts and brain. Improve function, reduce and eliminate aches and pains. Enjoy your life using your amazing living machinery!

2. When your body parts feel better, you will use them more. When you use them more, your body creates extra muscle, thicker bones, higher metabolism and you get leaner!

3. By practicing this 10-minute system, you create a healing and more energetic state.

1. Restoring and Maintaining Muscle Balance

Remember the example of the suspension bridge in Part One? If you tighten the cables on one side of the bridge, it becomes lopsided and causes structural problems. If that bridge could talk, it would moan and groan.

The same principle applies to your body. If you excessively tighten the cables on one side of your "body bridge" (bones and joints), that causes three main problems:

1. Makes your "body bridge" lopsided.
2. Causes structural problems, increasing the likelihood of joint damage.
3. Since our body can't talk, it complains with symptoms like aches, pains, strains, stiffness and swelling.

On the other hand, by improving muscle balance, we can:
1. *reduce and eliminate unpleasant symptoms,*
2. *improve function and*
3. *create more stable, long-lasting joints.*

Improving muscle balance also creates better energy transmission for our nerves (which are like electricity lines for our muscles). It's a good thing to give these lines space! If you ever pinched a nerve, then you know firsthand how that can cause tingling, numbness and pain.

Improved Blood Flow

Improving muscle balance improves blood flow as well. That's important because blood provides power to your muscles and brain so they can feel and function better. Improved circulation sends a signal to body parts telling them there is more power and stability. Then they can turn down and turn off symptoms like aches, pains, stiffness and swelling.

For example, when clients come to me with body pain, I help them create better blood flow to the area that hurts (they never practice a position that is painful). By improving blood flow, aches and pains lessen and even disappear.

Blood provides power to our muscles similar to hydraulic fluid providing power to a crane (not the bird). Without hydraulic fluid, that crane won't pick up cars at the junkyard. Blood also provides oxygen, nutrients and water, and takes away waste products. The famous psychiatrist and brain researcher Dr. Daniel Amen actually states, "improving blood blow is the fountain of youth" in his book *Magnificent Mind at Any Age*.[1]

Decreased Blood Flow
The circulatory system moves blood throughout your body with flexible pipelines (veins and arteries). When you have excessively tight and imbalanced muscles, that restricts this delivery system and the body complains.

You've experienced the difference blood flow can make in your daily life. Just think about how you feel after sitting in a car or plane for four hours. After being trapped like this, you've probably noticed how your overall body suffers. Plus, we usually don't drink enough water when we travel. Dehydration also negatively affects blood flow.

Decreased blood flow increases aches, pains and injury potential. It causes problems for brain function as well!

Now compare those post-four-hour sitting sensations to how your body feels after dancing for just 20 minutes (with a fully water-hydrated body). As a result, blood flow dramatically improves to your body parts and brain and you feel way better! It's not a fair

1. Daniel Amen, *Magnificent Mind at Any Age* (New York: Harmony Books, 2008), 16

competition. Dancing also forces the brain to coordinate intricate body movements, which means it is great brain training and stimulation.

2. Restoring and Maintaining Effective Joint Range of Motion

I get it—this title may not sound sexy. But let me assure you, your joints are amazing and worth discussing. They enable us to move and use our bodies with precision and complexity.

Question: What allows our joints to have effective range of motion?
Answer: Muscles

Question: What is effective joint range of motion?
Answer: That will be demonstrated for a variety of joints in Part Three. These include the feet, ankles, knees, hips, shoulders, wrists and spine (which contains a long series of interconnected joints that have a big impact on back and neck muscles).

Question: Why does the Jiffy Body system enable better functioning joints?
Answer: Because you learn how to activate and stretch muscles that will enable your joints **to have effective range of motion.**

Question: Why is it important to have effective joint range of motion?
Answer: With effective joint range of motion, you are way more likely to 1) use your joints and supporting muscles without

pain, and 2) maintain your joints **for the long haul** and prevent injuries.

Question: How long will this take?
Answer: With 10 minutes of daily practice, you can improve blood circulation, muscle balance, joint range of motion and lubrication. Also, did I mention you can practice this system in your pajamas?

The Long Haul: Joint Longevity

When your joints lack effective range of motion and stability, they wear out more quickly. Then you are more likely to have aches, pains, injuries and eventually surgery. Perhaps you may be concerned about the longevity of your hips and knees and the possibility of a joint replacement?

To prevent this, it's important to identify any of your joints that may currently lack effective range of motion. Here's an example: Let's say you can't bend your knee completely because your thigh muscles are too tight. Imagine how that would also disrupt the function of other joints in your ankles, feet, hips and even lower back. They would all struggle to compensate for that imbalance, become more injury-prone and likely wear out faster.

Sometimes the lack of range of motion in our joints is much less noticeable. **This system will help you identify and improve those joints before they become more noticeable problems for themselves and other joints and muscles.**

Better Shock Absorbers

A flexible supporting cast of muscles creates better shock absorption for your joints. Imagine if that suspension bridge we discussed earlier, decided to go for a walk. It would quickly break into pieces because there would be nothing to absorb the shock and impact of movement. Our body structures are lucky because we have muscles which absorb shock as we move. For example, when you walk or run, it's a lot more "cushiony" to land on feet with pliable foot and calf muscles. For this reason, you will practice creating flexible joint-specific muscles.

So Why Bother?

The consequences of neglecting to take simple, easy actions to benefit joints and muscle balance compound as we age. Have you ever seen someone struggle to walk down the street because their "body bridge" looks so lopsided? They have rounded shoulders, a hump in their upper back and their head faces down. This is an extreme example of both muscle imbalance and lost joint range of motion.

The combination of those two leads to decreased blood flow and loss of muscle mass. The more imbalanced you are, the harder it is to move. Therefore, you use your muscles less and the decreased demand allows them to shrink. **Smaller muscles put less pressure on your bones, which means they lose density, as well.**

On the flip side, by practicing and maintaining joint range of motion and muscle balance, you can move and use your body better.

For example, a client who is in his 80s and rides his horse three times a week told me **he has noticed getting up and down from the floor has become much easier since he has been practicing the Jiffy Body system. He also described how when he used to walk, it felt like a cable was pulling his body toward the ground. With daily joint range of motion and muscle balance practice, he now walks without any restriction.**

3. Identifying and Improving Weak Points, and Preventing Injuries

We all have our own personalized sets of strengths and weaknesses. I help clients identify their own combinations by running them through this system. As you practice, you might discover obvious weak points and those that are more subtle. It's especially valuable to discover the weak points you didn't know about!

Injury Prevention

For example, it's a lot better to discover that you have limited ankle range of motion before you put pressure on it by playing tennis. By identifying and improving weak points, you improve your ability to handle ballistic, unplanned-for life events like tripping on a turned-up rug, pothole, curb or ice.

One client of mine was unloading a moving truck and the driver drove off while she was still in the back of it. She had to jump out of the truck and land on her feet onto the asphalt. But she was not injured! She told me there was no way she would have handled it so well if she hadn't been practicing the Jiffy Body system.

By improving your weak points, you can feel and function way better! A piano teacher once told me, "When you're trying to learn a song, practice the parts of it that you can't play. That way you improve faster."

It's the same with weak point practice for your body. For example, one client sustained a horse-riding accident that severely limited hip range of motion on her left side. She also had excessively tight hamstrings that created back problems. First, she became comfortable practicing the entire system every day. Then she also practiced improving her weak points with an extra 5 to 10 minutes each day. Her back, hips, legs and upper body progressively felt a lot better. This also included a dramatically reduced incidence of leg cramps at night!

Feel Better, Use Your Body More, Get Leaner

You can lose weight and get leaner with this system! When you create more effective joints and improve muscle balance, it's easier to move and use your body. Increased body use causes muscle fiber growth. More muscle fiber creates a host of benefits including:

- Makes you a better calorie-burning machine, facilitating weight loss and, most importantly, becoming leaner.

- Improves blood circulation, which enhances nutrient delivery, detoxification, increased energy and feeling better in your body and brain.

- Puts more pressure on your leg and hip bones as well, thereby increasing bone density.

In fact, our bodies are living machinery. When we move, we maintain and can even upgrade our machinery. When we don't, we downgrade.

Have Some Fun!

That doesn't mean, however, that you have to work out for hours in the gym. You can obtain these benefits by first practicing this system. Make your body feel better and then you can use it more throughout your day.

Fun activities count, like going for a walk, gardening, and being active with your family and friends. Dancing is brain-stimulating and great range of motion practice for all of your joints. Doing your chores is also a great option. **Remember, joints are maintained for the long haul by using them in normal ranges of motion.** For example, raking leaves, picking weeds, vacuuming, cleaning dishes, dusting, sweeping and doing laundry all require different combinations of muscles and joint ranges of motion.

All those combinations benefit joint health and overall body function. As a result, you maintain your living machinery. That way you can continue using it with such interesting variations. As an added bonus you could "Tom Sawyer" your family members and convince them to chip in because chores are good for them!

You may notice that by sprinkling more bits of movement throughout the day, you feel more energetic and clear-headed! That happens because every time you move and use your muscles, you increase blood flow. That improves detoxification as well as nutrient and oxygen delivery. Just make sure that as you increase movement, you stay hydrated by drinking water.

The benefits of increasing your daily activity is not a radical concept. Before smart watches, there were pedometers designed to track your daily number of steps. Nowadays there are a variety of fitness tracking technologies. They report to you how much you actually move during the day. If the watch tells you that you aren't moving enough, then you can slowly increase.

I have had innumerable clients get leaner, lose weight, fit into their clothes and feel a ton better by taking the following simple actions:

- Tune up their body with the Jiffy Body system (so their body feels better and can better handle increased use).

- Track their activity and make a commitment to use their body more.

- Support their body by eating healthy, whole foods and avoiding processed foods. These include sugar, bread, chips, soda, crackers and juice (usually foods that are sold in a box, wrapper, bottle or bag).

No Brain, No Gain
When you increase your activity level, don't follow the worn-out cliché, "No Pain, No Gain." Many times, people try to force rapid improvement and endure aches, pains and even injury just to lose weight. You have a much better chance of handling increased

body demand when you strategically plan for small, incremental improvements over time.

Exercise

You may actually enjoy exercise! However, it can be hard to continue when you struggle with muscle imbalance, unstable joints and disgruntled body parts. For example, a number of my clients have been injured in their favorite yoga classes. This system helps you tune up your mechanical parts. When you combine that with a more patient, long-term approach to exercise, your body has a much better chance of handling activities you love!

Create a Healing and More Energetic State

As we rush through our days trying hard to get everything done, we often spend our time in a stressed fight-or-flight (sympathetic) state. A variety of factors contribute to this state including: lack of sleep, caffeine, refined sugars and not drinking enough water or eating quality whole foods. This makes it harder for the body to enter a healing state (parasympathetic).

This stressed environment is closely linked with adrenal fatigue, where the adrenal glands produce too much cortisol (a stress hormone). When the adrenals become so preoccupied with producing cortisol, they can then produce less of the other important hormones, including testosterone, pregnenolone and estrogen (in varying amounts, depending on your gender). Those hormones are valuable for energy, recovery and feeling your best!

This system helps your body and brain get a break by creating a parasympathetic state which can reduce heart rate, blood pressure and cortisol production. **That's why after practicing for 10 minutes, you can notice a variety of benefits such as: increased energy, reduced stress, less brain fog and feeling more grounded.**

PART THREE

INSPECT YOUR PARTS

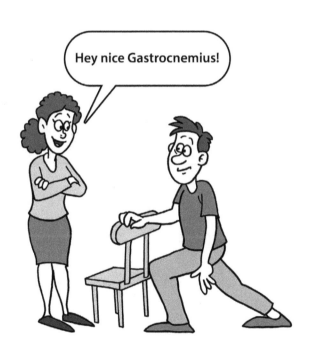

This section provides practice positions to benefit your feet, ankles, knees, hips, back, wrists, shoulders and neck. You will learn: 1) why we use these positions and 2) variations for most positions from easier to more challenging options (marked with a "+" sign).

Do not practice all of the positions at once.

That would take a lot longer than 10 minutes and is unnecessary! Go to Part Four when you are ready to practice. There you can start with "Practice Light" and learn how to safely implement this 10-minute system. **There are recommendations for how long to hold a stretch or how many repetitions to do for a range of motion position.**

Ankles and Feet

Balance starts on the ground floor where the **calf, tibialis and peroneus** muscles help to maintain balanced ankles and feet as well as ankle range of motion. When our feet and ankles are balanced, function improves up the ladder to the knees, hips and back. It's similar to a car's tires. They last longer and perform better when they are aligned with each other.

If one wheel is wobbly, that throws off the other wheels. Similarly, if any parts of your feet and ankles are "wobbly," that disrupts the knees, hips and lower back. Then these connecting parts have to work harder to stabilize you. Over time this increases the possibility of painful symptoms, dysfunction, injury and premature joint wear and tear.

Back of Lower Leg

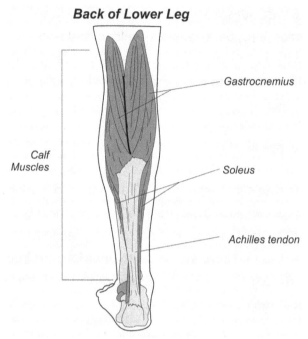

Gastrocnemius

Calf
Muscles

Soleus

Achilles tendon

Calf Muscles (Gastrocnemius and Soleus)
Besides being important for foot, ankle and knee stability, the Gastrocnemius and Soleus are also impressive words to use at a cocktail party. When these muscles are tight, they increase your chances of injury at the Achilles tendon (where they attach).

Tight calves disrupt your foot's ability to efficiently impact the ground. So why do people get tight calves? For starters, walking as an exercise is great. However, as you walk, your calves tighten to propel you forward. They tighten further by walking in high heels or any shoes where the heel is higher than the toes.

While you walk, you also balance the entire weight of your body on one side of calf muscles at a time with every step. They tighten again and again to counter that load. That's a ton of work!

When the calves are flexible, it's like walking in your favorite pair of sneakers. When the calves are tight, it's like walking in a new pair of stiff, leather shoes. As a result, you could notice other body parts complaining (feet, ankles, knees, hips, lower back). Pliable calf muscles absorb shock better for all of those parts. They also minimize impact and prevent injury to the Achilles tendon and your feet (including the commonly injured plantar fascia located on the bottom of your feet).

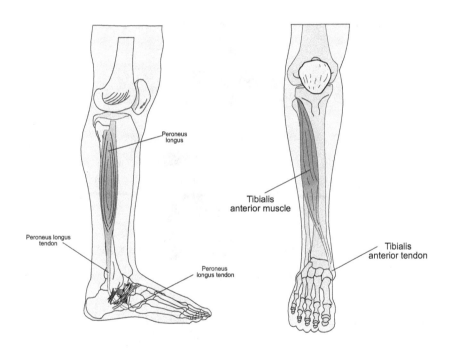

Peroneus Muscles and Tibialis Muscles

Both the peroneus (a group of three muscles) and the tibialis anterior connect from the side of your lower leg to points underneath both sides of your feet. That creates leverage for balancing the feet and ankles, resulting in better body balance and feet and ankle joint function.

If you were to trip on a toy and turn your ankle, the tibialis and peroneus muscles prevent the ankle from collapsing and creating injury and damage. They also support your foot's arch, creating a "cushioning" effect with every step. Since they absorb shock and create balance at the "ground floor," that benefits your knee, hip and lower back function as well. The tibialis allows your feet to point uphill and provides "brakes" when going downhill so you can stop. **That's a ton of benefits from a small group of muscles!**

Calves, Tibialis and Peroneus Practice Positions

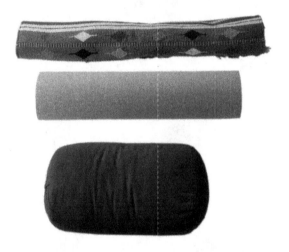

Using Props: Props are useful because they provide leverage to stretch the calves. They can include a yoga pillow (closest), rolled-up yoga mat or blanket.

You can practice the calf stretches in bare feet or socks (as long as you don't have any foot problems). That way, your feet will get to practice a little extra range of motion as they adjust to the contours of the prop. Make sure you have a clutter-free and softer practice space (such as a carpet).

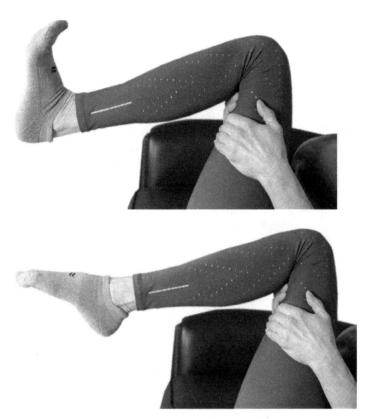

Toe Circles (A) and (B) (Peroneus and Tibialis Muscles):
Slightly recline in an armchair or couch. Pull one leg toward the chest
while holding the hands against the back of the thigh, below the knee.
To activate tibialis and peroneus muscles, draw a slow, complete circle
with the toes, starting at 12 o'clock (A). Then move the toes to 6 o'clock
(B) and then continue around to 12 o'clock again (A).

Go slowly and try to draw a full circle. If you rush, you won't fully activate
the tibialis and peroneus muscles, and this will minimize the benefit.
If you start to feel ankle or foot soreness, draw a smaller circle until you
feel no discomfort. Remember to draw circles in both directions. If you
notice soreness afterward, it's okay to take a day (or days) off from
practicing this position. That same principle goes for every position.

If it's difficult to draw a slow, complete circle, that means you have
identified a weak point. That's valuable to know! With consistent practice,
you will draw better circles. That creates better-balanced and more
stable feet, ankles, knees and hips!

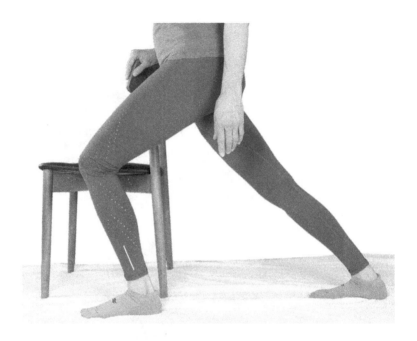

Straight Leg Calf Stretch (Gastrocnemius):
Stand next to a wall or chair in case you lose balance. Move one leg back and place that foot flat on the floor (back leg). Remember to keep that leg straight. Move the opposite leg forward and bend the knee, but not so far that it goes over the toes.

To increase the stretch on the back leg, 1) move the front foot forward and 2) keep the back leg straight. If you still don't feel enough stretch, then try the "+" version of this position. To decrease the stretch, place both legs closer together.

Try to keep the back foot in line with the ankle, knee and hip. That may be challenging to do if you tend to walk with your feet turned out or turned in, so don't force it. Just do what your body will comfortably allow. Over time, this can help create better alignment and function as you stand and move.

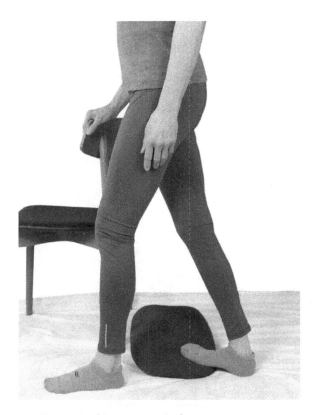

Straight Leg Calf Stretch+ (Gastrocnemius):
Stand next to a wall or chair in case you lose balance. Move one leg back and place the front part of that foot **against a prop** (back leg). Remember to keep the leg straight. Move the opposite leg forward and bend the knee, but not so far that it goes over the toes.

To increase the stretch on the back leg, 1) move the front foot forward and 2) keep the back leg straight. To decrease the stretch, place both legs closer together.

Try to point the back foot straight ahead in line with the ankle, knee and hip. That may be challenging to do if you tend to walk with your feet turned out or turned in, so don't force it. Just do what your body will comfortably allow. Over time, this can help create better alignment and function as you stand and move.

Notice the back foot and ankle joint point upward so you practice joint range of motion at the same time! Remember we practice range of motion to maintain our joints long term and improve daily function. For example, that particular foot angle is useful when walking uphill.

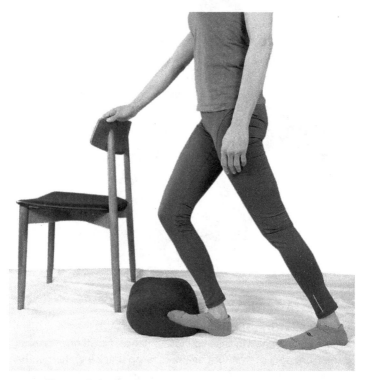

Bent Leg Calf Stretch (Soleus):
Stand next to a wall or chair for balance. Move one leg forward, bend the knee and place the front part of that foot against a prop (front leg). The knee of the back leg is slightly bent for stability.

To increase the stretch on the front leg, further bend the front knee. To decrease the stretch, bend the front knee less, or use a shorter prop to reduce the incline of the front foot.

Try to point the front foot straight ahead in line with the ankle, knee and hip. That may be challenging to do if you tend to walk with your feet turned out or turned in, so don't force it. Just do what your body will comfortably allow. Over time, this can help create better alignment and function as you stand and move.

As with the Gastrocnemius stretch, the foot against the prop is pointing "uphill" so you benefit by practicing ankle range of motion at the same time.

Knees, Hips and Lower Back

Knees

Our knees bend and straighten while we move. When they are forced to dramatically exceed this range of motion, knee injuries are more likely. Combinations of leg muscles keep our knees on track, so they stay within their intended range of motion. These muscles include hamstrings, quadriceps, adductors, glutes (indirectly), tibialis, peroneus and calf muscles.

Back of Leg **Front of leg**

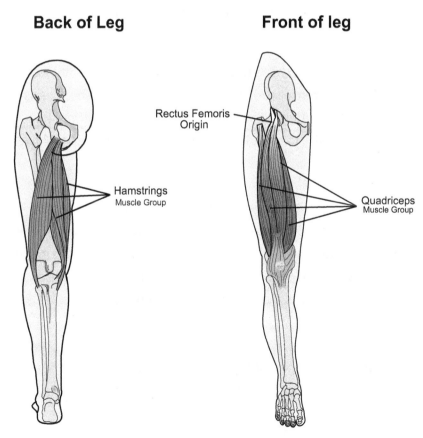

Rectus Femoris
Origin

Hamstrings
Muscle Group

Quadriceps
Muscle Group

Hamstrings Muscles:
The hamstrings are a group of three muscles on the upper back of your legs. Notice the attachments on both sides of the knee. For this reason, the hamstrings have leverage to stabilize your knees and create better balance when you move.

Quadriceps Muscles:
The quadriceps are a group of four muscles on the upper front of your legs. They are important knee stabilizers, and along with your butt muscles, provide power for:
— Getting up from the floor or a chair.
— Climbing stairs or a hill.

To stay good at these activities, then practice them (within your comfort zone!). When you use muscles, your body builds muscle fiber. That's positive because these fibers are like motors that enable you to keep using your amazing living machine! Muscle fibers put pressure on bones as well, causing them to thicken.

Tight quadriceps and hamstrings restrict your knees' ability to bend and straighten, disrupting efficient movement. Before meeting Sean, I had super tight hamstrings, despite years of effort to stretch them out. That resulted in restricted movement and lower back pain.

With the following techniques (on pages 60-61), I consistentlyl consistently improved hamstring flexibility and back function. So, if there's hope for me, that's a good sign for others who might say, "That's just my genetics. I've always been tight." Sean used to say that, "Genetics are a predisposition, not a sentence."

Flat Back
Excessively tight hamstrings create downward pressure on the back side of the pelvis. That can cause the lower back arch to

flatten (flat back) and the butt to curve under and disappear. When you are out in public, take some time to look at people's butts (yes, that sounds peculiar). You will recognize this muscle imbalance where some people have very little butt and very little lower back arch.

When the butt muscles are in this disadvantageous position, they lose power. That is important because the butt muscles stabilize your hips and knees and they are the foundation for the lower back.

Sway Back
Problems can also happen for the lower spine when the quadriceps muscles are excessively tight. That creates downward pressure on the front side of the pelvis. This can cause the lower back arch to increase excessively (sway back).

Many of my clients have eliminated lower back pain and improved movement and hip function by creating a balance of flexibility between their quadriceps and hamstrings. We are a symphony of joints and muscles working together so we can move freely and enjoy our bodies.

Front of Legs

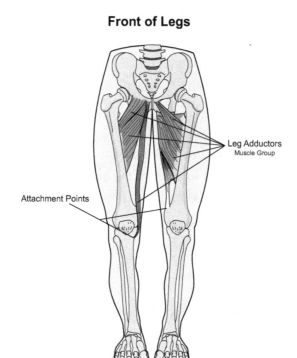

Adductor Muscles:
Because the leg adductor muscles overlap, they are shown on both legs. That way you can see all five of these muscles at once. Notice the attachment points for two of the muscles close to the knee, providing leverage to stabilize this joint.

Knees and Hips

The adductor muscles stabilize both the knees and hips. They help the knees stay in their intended range of motion (primarily to bend and straighten). For example, the adductors keep both the knees and hips stable when you trip, move sideways, dance or play sports (where side-to-side movement is important). When the adductors aren't doing their job, the knees are more likely to sustain pain, injury and dysfunction.

Excessively tight adductors restrict hip range of motion, and that's a bad thing for pain-free function and long-term hip health. In addition, creating flexible adductors can allow more blood flow to your groin, and this contributes to a healthy, happy sex life.

Over time, as you stretch these muscles, it's most ideal to notice equal tension on both legs. Otherwise, your "body bridge" can be pulled off-balance, disrupting the function of the hips, pelvis and spine.

Back of Legs

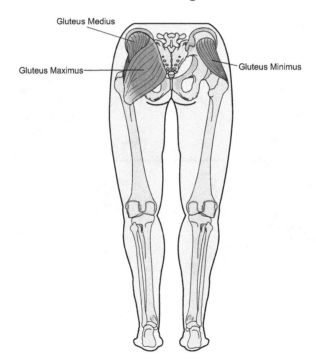

Gluteus Medius

Gluteus Maximus

Gluteus Minimus

Glutes (Butt Muscles):
The glutes coordinate with the adductors to provide hip and knee stability.
There are three layers of glute muscles: maximus, medius and minimus.
Because these muscles overlap, they are shown here using both legs
so you can see all of them at once.

Excessively tight glute muscles restrict hip range of motion, which is a bad thing for long-term hip health (as well as for the health of your knees, ankles and feet). As you stretch these muscles over time, you will want to notice balanced tension on both legs to help create a better-balanced "body bridge" and improved function.

Quadriceps, Hamstrings, Adductors and Glutes Practice Positions

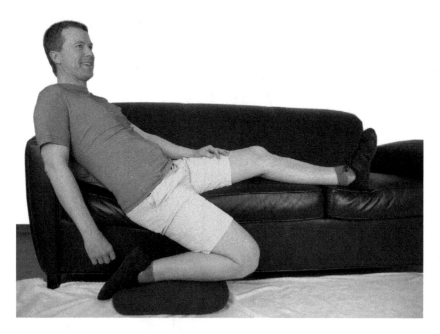

Quadriceps Couch Stretch:
Sit sideways on a couch. Put a pillow under the lower back for support so you can comfortably lean against the armrest. The upper leg is supported lengthwise on the couch. Pull the lower leg back. Support that foot and ankle on a pillow or prop (as demonstrated in the photo). Slightly recline until you feel a stretch in the quadriceps of the lower leg.

As the lower leg drops down, you also practice hip range of motion on that side. One simple position creates lots of body benefit!

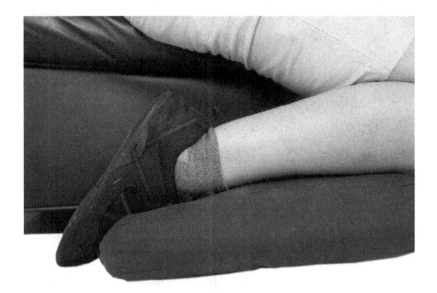

Quadriceps Couch Stretch Close-up of Ankle:
To reduce any discomfort you may feel in the ankle or foot:
1) slightly move the knee of the lower leg up and away from the floor;
2) keep a shoe on (as opposed to being barefoot); and
3) support the foot and ankle with a prop.

If either ankle is sore, your body is warning you of a weak point. To help the ankles improve, you will practice the previously described "Toe Circles" (in the section on Ankles and Feet). Toe Circles are included with each practice plan demonstrated in Part Four. Remember not to practice any position that is painful!

Notice that the ankle enables the bottom foot to point away from the shin. That way you practice ankle joint range of motion at the same time! Remember we practice range of motion to maintain our joints long term and improve daily function. That particular foot angle can also be useful when walking downhill.

Your Couch Is Useful

The couch is a great place to stretch the quadriceps. 1) You can keep the ankle in line with the knee and hip. When people try this stretch on the floor, they often pull their foot and ankle out to the side, which can twist and torque the knee. 2) You effectively stretch all of the quadriceps, including the rectus femoris. Notice in the quadriceps illustration (page 53) that the rectus femoris originates higher up on the pelvis. That gives it leverage to pull your leg toward your body (which is important for walking).

When this muscle is excessively tight, it pulls the pelvis downward, acting like a high-tension cable that pulls your "body bridge" off-center. As a result, that can impede movement and create hip and back problems.

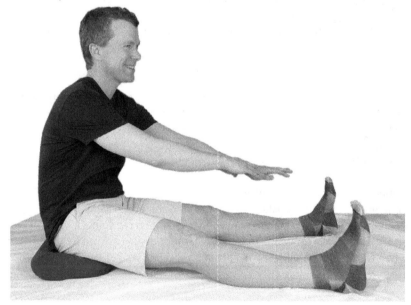

Hamstrings Stretch:
Sit near the edge of a prop (see page 48). Put your legs in a "V" straight in front of you. Lean toward one foot with an upright upper body. You'll feel

a stretch on the same side, down the leg and even into the calves. Your knee may buckle up to release the pressure of the stretch. As you improve over time, you'll notice your knee relaxes more and buckles less.

To increase the stretch, lean further toward one foot while keeping the upper body upright and the leg straight. To decrease the stretch, release away from the foot.

You may be tempted to fold over like a rag doll so you can reach further. However, that diverts the stretch more to the lower back, which defeats the point of the stretch. By sitting upright and then reaching forward, you'll keep the pressure on the hamstrings.

It's easier to stay upright by sitting **toward the edge of a prop.** That creates leverage to get a better hamstring stretch. This can be especially helpful if your hamstrings are tight. You can also reach under the leg and rub the hamstrings while stretching them (which can help them relax).

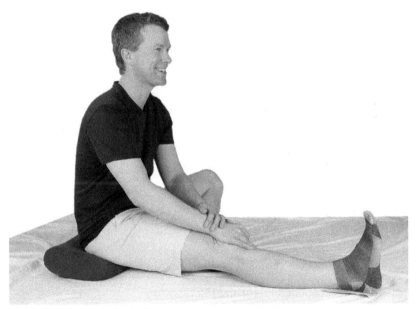

Hamstrings Stretch Single Leg+:
This option enables you to better isolate the hamstrings one side at a time. If you have any knee issues, pass on this position.

Sit near the edge of a prop (see page 48). Bend one knee and tuck the leg in toward your body. The opposite leg is straight out in front of you.

Lean toward the straight leg with an upright upper body. Lean further forward to increase and less forward to decrease the stretch.

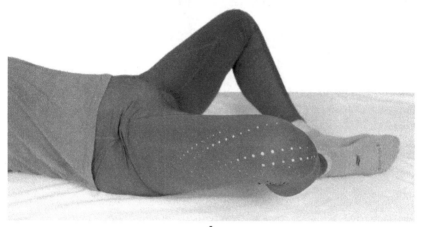

A

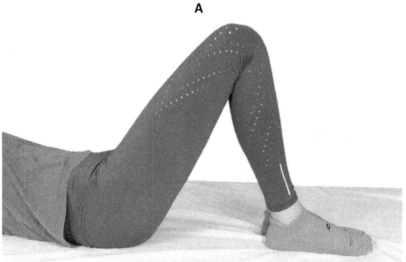

B

Butterfly Stretch (Adductors) (A) and (B):
The adductors, in particular, can be super sensitive, so it's a good idea to warm them up before stretching. That increases blood flow and makes them more pliable. Alternate between Position A and B up to 20 times to warm them up. You can do less, as well, if this feels challenging. After the warm-up repetitions, allow the legs to stretch and rest in position (A). You stretch the adductors and at the same time practice hip range of motion.

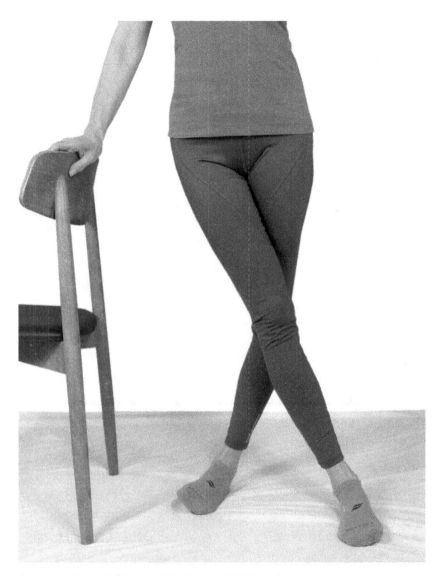

Crossover Stretch (Gluteus Medius and Minimus):
Stand next to a wall or chair and hold on for balance. Cross the right leg over the left, placing more body weight on the left leg. Then slowly let the left hip move sideways and away from the body until you feel a stretch on the outside of that leg. Then try stretching the opposite side with left over right, and the right hip moves sideways and away from the body.

Hip Range of Motion

In Colorado, people sometimes joke that the great thing about 4-wheel drive is it enables you to get stuck in the snow higher up in the mountains. Similarly, our hips are high performers. They are a ball-and-socket joint (like the shoulders), enabling amazing diversity including going up and down stairs, moving sideways, dancing and playing.

The hips can have problems, as well, if you don't practice or use enough hip range of motion. For this reason, the muscles that keep your hips stable can become weak and dysfunctional. That can lead to pain and possible injuries (not to mention the increased likelihood of an eventual hip replacement).

On the other hand, by practicing hip range of motion, you create several benefits: 1) you spread the lubricant synovial fluid in the joint (lubrication promotes joint longevity), 2) facilitate movement, and 3) prevent injuries.

You will also learn to stretch a variety of hip-related muscles which improves shock absorption, promotes hip joint longevity and facilitates movement. Imagine Sean's excitement when clients were able to avoid hip surgery by using these techniques.

Back of Legs

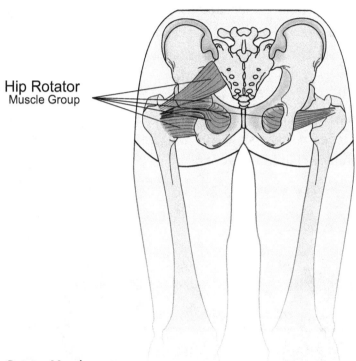

Hip Rotator
Muscle Group

Hip Rotator Muscles:
These six hip muscles rotate the hip and leg away from your middle.
They are a deep layer of muscles that attach from your pelvis to the top of
your leg bones. As a result, they have leverage to keep the ball of your hip
joint stable in the socket. They also enable effective joint range of motion.
That's important for pain-free, long-term hip use!

The hips and supporting muscles are highlighted in this book because they
are so heavily used for all movement. For this reason, there are a variety
of positions for practicing 1) hip range of motion and 2) hip-related muscle
flexibility. Many clients have told me they've noticed improved hip function
by practicing and improving these two categories.

Hip Rotators and Hip Flexibility Practice Positions

When you practice, don't use all of the hip positions shown here.
There are variations demonstrated from easier to more challenging.
That way as you practice, you can choose the options that work
best for your body. When you are ready to practice, go to
Part Four: Let's Practice!

**If you have had hip surgery, do not practice the hip rotators or
hip stretches in this system. You will need to get a specific
maintenance plan from your doctor.**

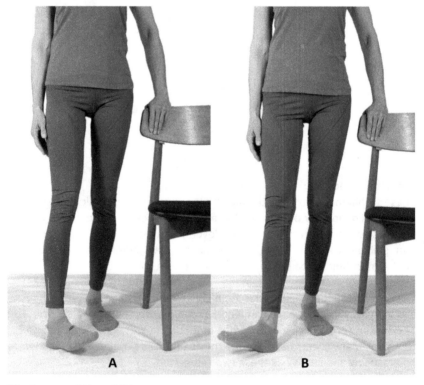

A   B

Hip Rotators (A) and (B):
Stand next to a wall or chair and hold on for balance. Rest your body weight
mostly on one leg. The opposite leg is slightly forward of the standing leg,

balanced on the heel. Rotate that leg first toward the middle and then away from the middle, as in pictures (A) and (B). Rotate the leg as far as it will go in each direction with comfort.

Go slow and easy and don't force either direction!
Remember, this is not a workout! It's supposed to be easy. By practicing range of motion, you lubricate the hip and create joint stability. It's also a great hip warm-up to use before any more strenuous leg activity.

To ensure that the hip muscles are rotating the leg, try this experiment. Put your hand on the hip muscles of the rotating leg. You should feel muscles in that area contracting and relaxing as the leg rotates back and forth.

The Hip Rotator Challenge+
You can make the hip rotator more challenging: 1) You don't hold on to a chair or wall. However, it's still a good idea to stand next to one in case you lose your balance. 2) The standing leg (the one holding more of your body weight) is straight (no bend in the knee).

This combination forces hip muscles on the standing leg to work harder. Place your hand on the hip of the standing leg and you'll feel those hip muscles contracting while the opposite leg rotates.

This is great hip practice! The standing leg's hip muscles practice stabilizing the hip joint, while the opposite leg's hip muscles practice rotation. These essential hip skills enable efficient movement and long-term function.

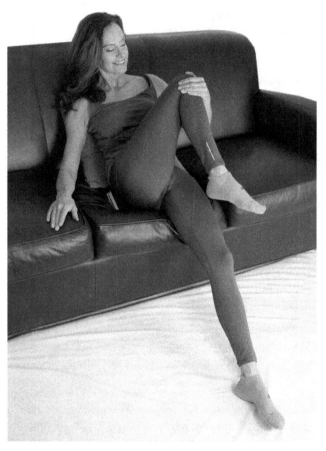

Hip Stretch (Couch):
Recline back in a couch. Place a pillow underneath your lower back for support. Place a hand on the outside of one knee. Then slowly pull that leg across the middle of the body, angling the leg toward the opposite side's shoulder. If you want more stretch, pull the knee closer to the opposite shoulder. For less stretch, release the leg away from the shoulder.

This may look similar to the iliopsoas stretch on the couch where you pull the leg in a straight line toward your body (page 74). The difference is that now you pull the leg across at an angle. That way you stretch your gluteus maximus (page 57) and external hip rotator muscles (page 65). Both the couch and chair (next position) are great options for stretching hip muscles because they enable you to easily adjust the degree of stretch. At the same time, you are practicing hip range of motion!

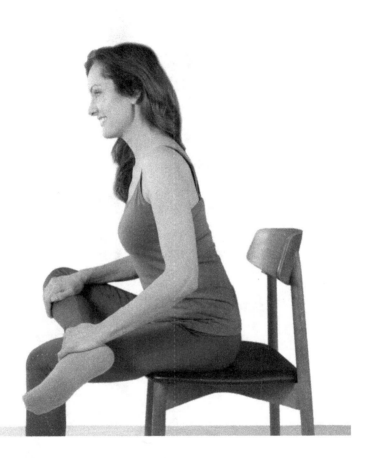

Cross Leg Hip Stretch (Chair):
This position is usually uncomfortable if you already have any knee soreness. In that case, use "Hip Stretch (Couch)" instead. Otherwise, sit upright in a chair. Lift one leg and rest the side of that ankle on top of the opposite leg. You may already feel a stretch. If not, then keep the upper body upright and slowly lean forward. Try not to flop down and over at the waist. That causes the stretch to move from the hip to the lower back instead.

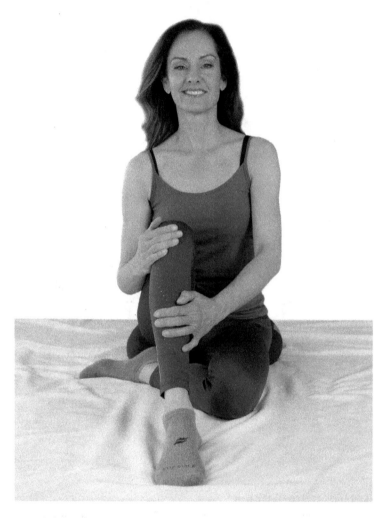

Hip Stretch (Floor)+:
This is a more advanced hip stretch. Only use this position if you are able to easily practice the other hip positions.

Sit toward the edge of a prop on the floor (see page 48). The prop makes it easier to sit upright. Bend the right knee. Pull that leg slightly toward the chest. Then place the heel of the right foot flat on the floor. Slide the left leg underneath the right until you feel a hip stretch. After that, try the opposite side.

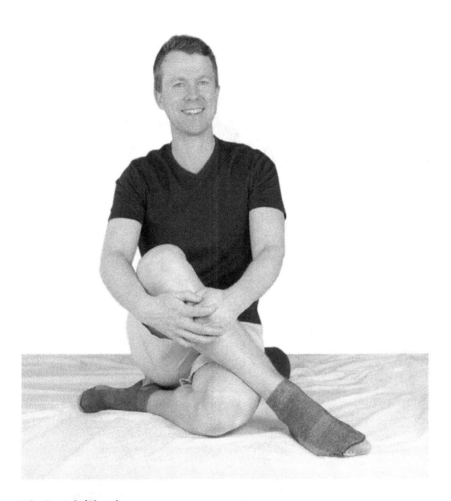

Hip Stretch (Floor)++:
To make Hip Stretch Floor+ more challenging, move the right leg around the left knee (as in the picture). Make sure to sit upright. If you slouch over, you decrease the hip stretch and create more of a lower back stretch instead. Remember to stretch both sides.

Back Health and Spinal Range of Motion

Front of Legs and Spine

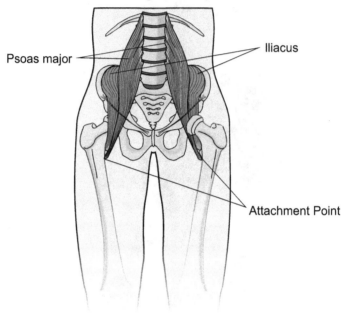

Psoas major

Iliacus

Attachment Point

Iliopsoas Muscle:
The iliopsoas connects from both sides of the spine and attaches at the
upper part of both leg bones. For this reason, when you stretch
the iliopsoas, you usually feel it in that upper, inside part of each leg.

The iliopsoas tightens to pull your legs up while walking. It also
tightens while sitting. The more you sit, the more the iliopsoas
gets good at holding that shortened position. You may have
noticed that it is harder to stand up straight and walk after a
sitting session. That is because now your shortened iliopsoas
is working against you!

For example, a client in his 80s told me he was having a hard time standing up straight while walking. Teaching him how to create a more flexible iliopsoas enabled him to walk upright without issue.

In addition, a shortened iliopsoas can cause structural problems for your "body bridge." For example, another client consulted me because of recurring back and hip pain stemming from an accident. She dramatically improved by practicing iliopsoas flexibility and the Jiffy Body system. She even gets compliments on her posture from people at the exercise classes she attends.

A flexible iliopsoas can prevent nerve impingement and improve shock absorption for your spine. It allows easier movement, can eliminate lower back pain symptoms and prevent injuries. The iliopsoas is so important, I've included several ways to stretch it.

Iliopsoas Practice Positions

When you begin to practice in Part Four, you will only use one version of the iliopsoas positions that are demonstrated here. You will start with the easiest option for every position. Do not practice all of the different options now.

If you have had hip surgery, do not practice the iliopsoas stretches in this system (which also stretch your hips). You will need to get a specific maintenance plan from your doctor.

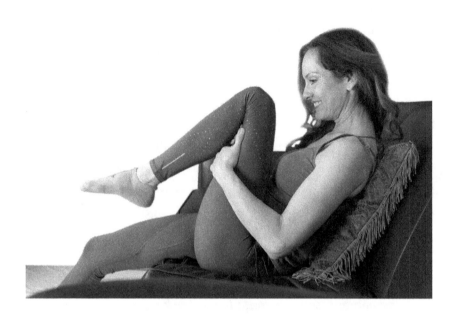

Wishbone Stretch (Couch):
Sit near the edge of the couch. Slightly lift one leg and place your hands on the bottom side of the leg, below the knee. This hand position is useful if you have any knee soreness (as opposed to placing your hands on top of the upper shin).

Recline until the upper body is supported by the back of the couch. For extra support and comfort, you can also put a pillow behind your back.

Pull the upper leg toward the chest. The lower leg is straight out in front of you. To decrease the stretch, release the upper leg away from the chest. To increase the stretch, pull the upper leg closer to the chest.

Make sure you are very comfortable with the wishbone stretch on the couch before trying any of the more advanced iliopsoas stretches! Remember, when you are ready to practice go to Part Four.

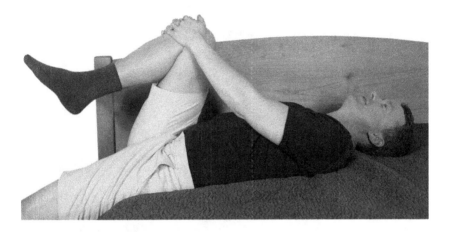

Wishbone Stretch (Bed)+:

Sit near the edge of a bed. Then slightly lift one leg and place your hands on the bottom side of the leg, below the knee. This hand position is useful if you have any knee soreness (as opposed to placing your hands on top of the upper shin as in this picture).

Slowly lean back onto the bed and pull the leg toward the chest. The lower leg is straight out in front of you. To decrease the stretch, release the upper leg away from the chest. To increase the stretch, pull the upper leg closer to the chest.

Doing this stretch on a bed gives you more leverage than the couch to pull the legs away from each other (like a wishbone). With all of these iliopsoas stretches, you practice hip range of motion at the same time, which benefits long-term hip joint health as well!

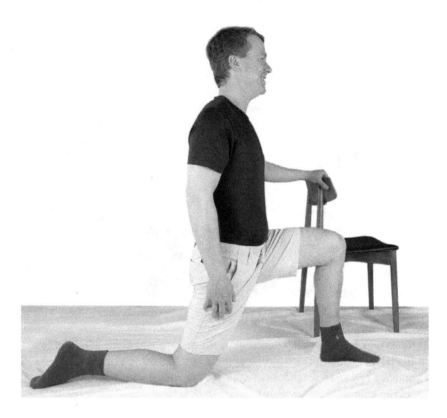

Wishbone Stretch (Floor)+:
Kneel on the floor. Place your left hand on a couch or chair for balance. Step forward with the left leg and keep the upper body upright.

Place the front foot flat on the floor. For more stretch, place the front foot further forward. For less stretch, place the front foot closer to your body.

Notice the rear leg moves back away from the body. That helps "unlock" the iliopsoas muscle and hip joints which can get stuck in a forward position while you sit at a desk or in a car.

Remember, the more hours you spend doing the same activities (like sitting), the more specific actions you need to take to counteract those activities (to avoid muscle imbalance and pain).

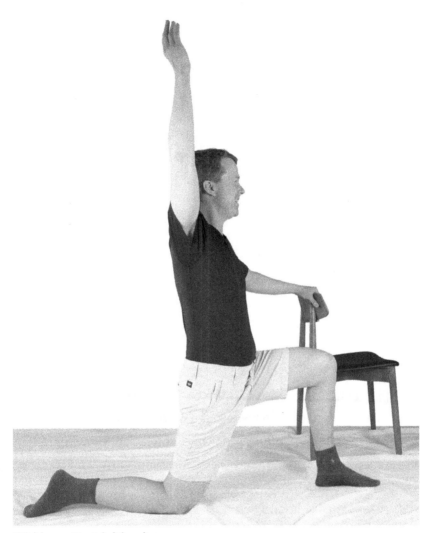

Wishbone Stretch (Floor)++:
Definitely don't try this position until you have easily practiced the other iliopsoas positions.

Kneel on the floor, with a folded towel or something soft under your knees.
Place your left hand on a couch or chair for balance. Step forward with the left leg and place the front foot flat on the floor. Raise the right arm and keep the upper body upright. For more stretch, place the left foot further forward. For less stretch, place the left foot closer to the body. Remember to stretch both sides and practice with the right foot forward as well.

Spinal Range of Motion

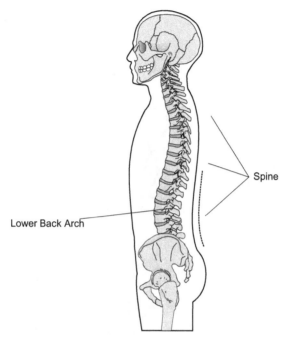

Our spine contains a series of interconnected joints. All of these individual joints need to have enough range of motion (mobility) for efficient spine function. When there is a lack of mobility at any point along the spine, that: 1) causes symptoms like aches and pains, 2) limits the ability to use your back with ease and 3) increases the likelihood of a back injury.

To avoid a "kink in the chain," you maintain and improve back and spine health by consistently practicing spinal range of motion. This includes sideways, rounding, arching, twisting and lengthening (within your comfort zone). With consistent practice, you can improve function, reduce aches and pains and facilitate real-world spine activities. These include sitting, standing and movement.

Even lying down on the ground or bed will be more comfortable when your spine has adequate mobility.

Lower Back Arch

The Romans used arches to build structures that still stand today. The lower back section of the spine uses an arch as well to disperse the jarring impact of movement and gravity (although the arch in the low back is not nearly as pronounced).

A) To get a sense of the lower back arch, sit on a flat chair and reach behind your back with one hand. Put it on the arch of your lower back (as long as that is comfortable for your shoulder). Then allow yourself to slouch and roll back more onto your butt muscles. As you do this, you will notice that the lower back arch flattens. When you sit on a couch or in an armchair, you will notice the same effect, and in fact, that it's hard to sit any other way.

B) To feel the opposite effect, once again sit on a flat chair, reach behind your back with one hand and put it on your lower back arch. This time roll forward onto your pelvis, away from your butt muscles. As you do this, you will notice the lower back arch increases. Gently roll back and forth a few times between A) and B) so you can feel the difference.

How you consistently sit can impact the lower back arch. If you roll back onto the butt muscles (like most people) and practice this position every day for hours and hours, over time the body builds the muscle patterns to accommodate that position. Then when you get up and walk around, you are more likely to take this muscle imbalance and a flattened lower back arch with you. This imbalance contributes to lower back aches, pains and dysfunction.

Spinal Range of Motion Practice Positions

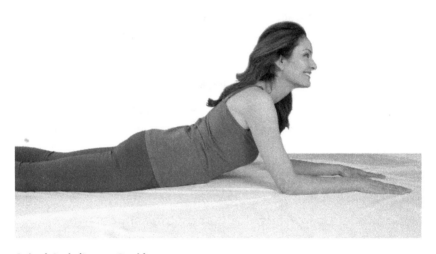

Spinal Arch (Lower Back):
This position can help counter the effects of excessive sitting with a flattened arch. Lie on the floor with your stomach down. Slide the elbows underneath your shoulders. Push the upper body away from the floor until you feel the arch accentuating in the lower back.

You may notice that this position is super easy because you already have plenty of lower back arch. If that's the case, then do not practice this position. Creating excessive arch could have a negative impact for your back health. You could occasionally check back and try this position just to make sure you are maintaining your arch.

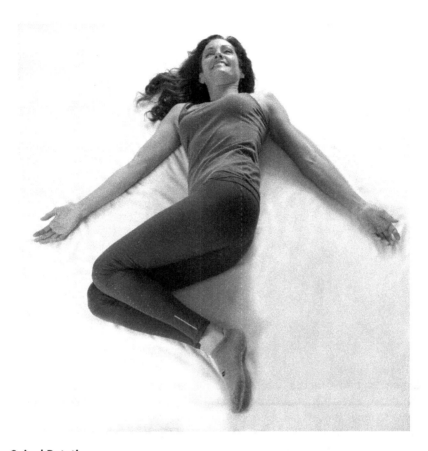

Spinal Rotation:

Lie on the floor, preferably on a carpet or yoga mat. Fold both legs to one side at about a 45-degree angle to the waist. You can use a pillow below the bottom side of the lower leg to make the stretch easier. Rest your arms at your sides on the floor. If that is uncomfortable, move your arms closer to the body or on top of your body.

To make the stretch more challenging, try stacking the top knee directly over the bottom knee. You can also bring your legs closer to a right angle with your body. To make the stretch easier, place the legs closer to a straight line with the body. Remember, start small, especially if you are new to practicing spinal rotation!

For recommendations on the length of time to hold a stretch, see *Part Four: Let's Practice!*

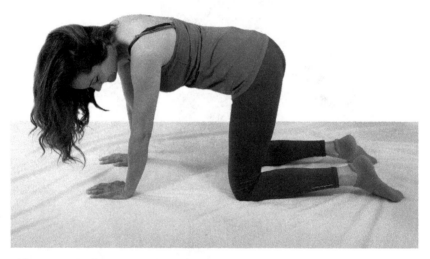

Sideways Spinal:
Get on "all fours" on the floor. Line up the hands slightly forward of the shoulders. Picture your body as an accordion. The head and left shoulder curve to meet the left hip. Then the right shoulder and head curve around to meet the right hip. Of course, our spine is not as flexible as an accordion, so don't expect as much range of motion.

Go back and forth slowly from side to side. By going more slowly, you are safer with your spine and you get more benefit. For recommendations on the number of repetitions, see *Part Four: Let's Practice!*

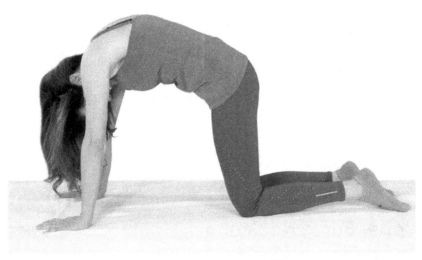

Round and Arch (Spine) (A)

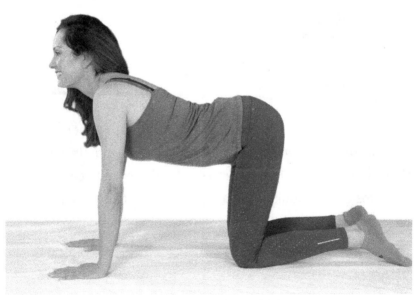

Round and Arch (Spine) (B)

Round and Arch (Spine) (A) and Round and Arch (Spine) (B)
Get on "all fours" on the ground. Line up your hands slightly in front
of the shoulders. A) Round the spine like a string is pulling it up toward
the ceiling. Allow the head to drop as the spine goes up. B) Then allow
the spine to move toward the floor, increasing the arch in the lower back.
As the arch increases, the head curls back up toward the ceiling.

Stay well within a comfortable range of motion as you alternate between
position (A) and (B). By going more slowly, you are safer with your spine
and get more benefit from each position.

Upper Back, Neck, Brain, Shoulders and Wrists

Have you ever noticed somebody whose shoulders and head are
too far forward, and they may have a hump in their upper back?
As mentioned in Part One, lots of sitting can be a major cause
for developing varying degrees of this imbalance (from hardly
noticeable to extreme).

A majority of people tend to sit with their head and shoulders too
far forward. The longer they sit without taking a muscle balance
break, the more likely they are to eventually experience structural
problems to the shoulders, head and neck, and also symptoms
like aches and pains.

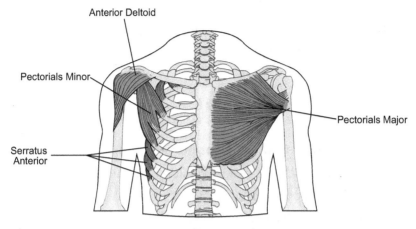

Upper Front Muscles

Excessively tightening cables on one side of a suspension bridge makes it lopsided and causes structural problems.

Similarly, sitting can cause excessively tight upper front "muscle cables" and our "body bridge" to become lopsided. That results in our structure (shoulders and neck) being pulled forward and off-balance. Gravity then has more leverage to pull us toward the ground. As a result of this structural imbalance, common symptoms occur with the shoulders, wrists, neck, elbows and upper back. These include pain, stiffness, blood flow restriction and nerve impingement.

Another unfortunate result of this muscle imbalance is a lack of coordination as you stand and move. If you walk with your head and shoulders too far forward, it's a lot harder to keep your balance! Even if your upper body frame is slightly off-center and too far forward, that negatively affects movement and coordination.

We can reverse this imbalance and feel a lot better in the process! **By stretching out the upper front "muscle cables,"** we allow our shoulders, upper back and neck to line up better with the rest of the body.

Upper Front Practice Positions

The following upper front positions provide variable degrees of difficulty starting with the easiest version first. Please remember not to do all of the positions now! When you are ready to practice, go to Part Four to pick a practice plan.

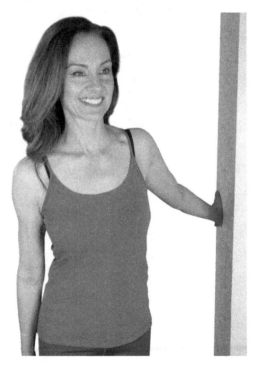

Upper Front Stretch (1):
Place a hand on a wall below the height of the shoulder. Then slightly rotate the upper body away from the wall. You should feel a stretch in the chest and shoulder. If this feels easy, you can increase the stretch by placing your hand higher on the wall (at shoulder height or slightly higher).

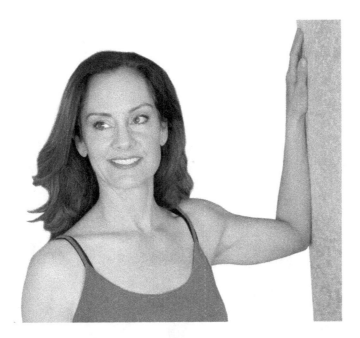

Upper Front Stretch (2)+:

Stand next to a wall. Place the underside of the hand, forearm and elbow against the wall. The elbow lines up slightly below the height of the shoulder. Gently rotate your body away from the wall until you feel a stretch. There are three options provided for the upper front stretch. (1) is the easiest and (2) and (3) are more challenging.

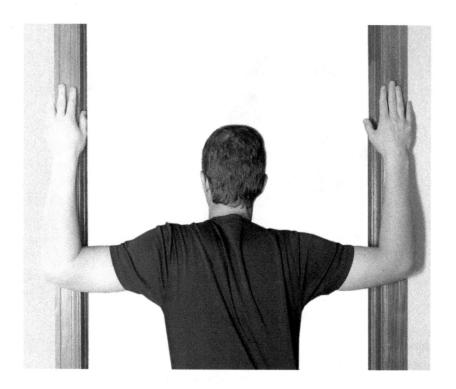

Upper Front Stretch (3)+:
Stand and face a door frame. Place the underside of your hands, forearms and elbows against the door frame. The elbows line up slightly below the height of the shoulders. Gently lean forward with the upper body until you feel a stretch.

To increase the stretch, lean further forward. To decrease the stretch, lean less far forward. Don't let the head drop. Instead, keep it in alignment with the upper body.

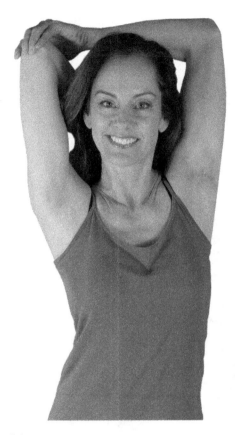

Reaching Elbow (1):
Slowly pull the elbow straight up and back toward the side of the head. To increase the stretch, pull the elbow closer to your head. To decrease the stretch, allow the elbow to release away from the head.

Your head may move forward as you pull the arm back. With consistent practice, it's easier to keep the head in line with the upper body. However, don't try to force it to stay upright. That could aggravate your neck.

You may also notice considerable tightness in the back of your upper arm (triceps muscle). With practice, you will progressively be able to pull your elbow up higher.

You benefit by releasing tight upper front muscles and practicing shoulder range of motion at the same time! Remember, practicing range of motion helps us maintain our joints for the long term. This particular range of motion position can also be useful when you are, for example, trying to pull a glass out of a cabinet.

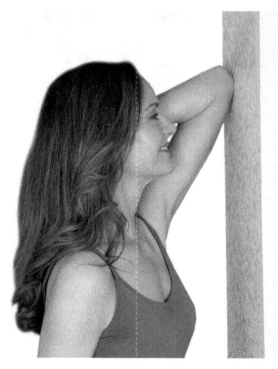

Reaching Elbow (2):

For some people, this is an easier option than Reaching Elbow (1). Stand and face a wall. Gently guide your elbow up until it rests against the wall at a point where you feel a comfortable stretch. To increase the stretch, place the elbow higher on the wall. To decrease the stretch, place the elbow lower on the wall.

Your head may move forward as your arm moves up and back. With consistent practice, it's easier to keep the head in line with the upper body. However, don't try to force the head to stay upright. That could aggravate your neck.

Upper Back Muscles

We just discussed how excessively tight upper front muscles pull the upper body structure forward and down toward the ground. Another effect of this muscle imbalance is that upper back muscles become overstretched. That causes them to stiffen and restrict blood flow.

Then several problems can occur: 1) soreness and pain for the shoulders, upper back and neck, 2) increased potential for injury to the shoulder and neck joints, and 3) restricted blood flow to the brain causing headaches and reduced mental energy.

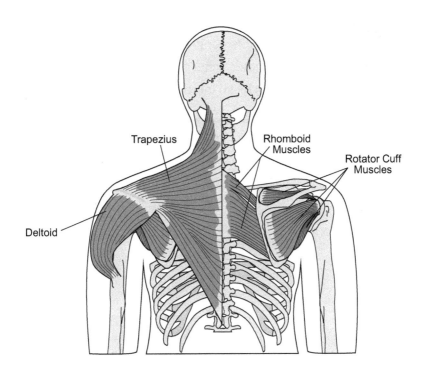

Upper Back Muscles

You can reverse this effect on your body frame by first stretching upper front muscles (as previously described). Then you activate and pump blood into the upper back muscles. That way they have more power to hold a position and prevent your "body bridge" from getting pulled forward.

Activated upper back muscles are the anchor that provides stability for the shoulders and arms every time you use them. If you have had shoulder, elbow and even wrist problems, one of the best things you can do is to activate these upper back muscles!

Restoring balance to your upper "body bridge" has three main benefits: 1) creates more stable, long-lasting neck and shoulder joints 2) reduces and eliminates aches and pains, and 3) improves blood flow to the brain which can increase mental energy and reduce or eliminate headaches.

Upper Back Practice Positions

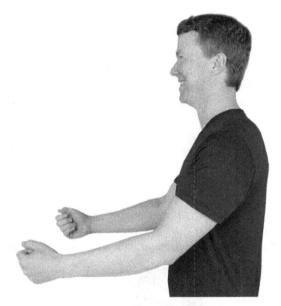

Row Boat (A)

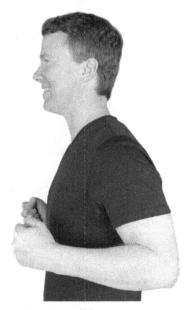

Row Boat (B)

Row Boat (A) and Row Boat (B):

(A) While standing, place your arms straight out in front of you like a forklift.
(B) Pull the arms back until you feel a contraction in the upper back muscles.
Then release back to position (A).

Sometimes the shoulders elevate toward the ears while doing Row Boat.
Instead, allow the shoulders to relax and keep the elbows at your side.
For the recommended number of repetitions, see *Part Four: Let's Practice!*

Make sure not to just swing the arms back and forth. You put the "mind
in the muscle" and squeeze the upper back muscles with every repetition.
As an experiment, ask a friend to put their hand on these muscles as you
pull back. That will give you a better feel for the muscles that are engaging.

Remember, this isn't a workout. This is a daily activity to pump blood
into upper back muscles. That way they can create better upper body
muscle balance and provide a foundation for your shoulders and head.

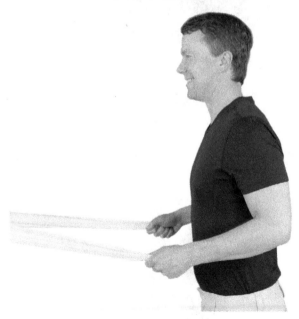

Row Boat+:

If you have a rubber resistance band, you can use that as well to alternate
between positions (A) and (B). Using resistance may make it easier to feel the
upper back muscles working.

Allow the shoulders to relax so they don't move up toward the ears. This position is not designed to make you huff and puff. This is a daily activity to activate upper back muscles so they can create better upper body muscle balance and provide a foundation for your shoulders, head and neck.

Shoulder Function and Range of Motion

The shoulders can have excellent range of motion because they are a ball-and-socket joint (like the hips). Your rotator cuff muscles stabilize this joint and enable effective range of motion. They are similar in function to the smaller hip rotator muscles that secure the hip joints (see page 65).

Look at your rotator cuff muscles. They are detailed in the upper back muscles illustration (see page 91). There is a fourth rotator cuff muscle as well that connects to the front side of the shoulder. Because of their location around the top of the arm bone, these muscles have leverage to stabilize the shoulder joint.

Wobbly Wheel

A wobbly wheel disrupts the other wheels on a car and prevents smooth driving. Similarly, the shoulder joint can become "wobbly" because of dysfunctional rotator cuff muscles. This creates problems for the other "wheels," including elbows, wrists, upper back and neck.

You create stable shoulder joints and benefit those other "wheels" by 1) creating better upper body muscle balance as presented on pages 84-94, and 2) training your rotator cuff muscles. For example, I've had numerous clients eliminate wrist and elbow problems by focusing on these two areas (as well as practicing wrist range of motion positions which are also included in this section).

If the following shoulder rotator cuff exercises (rotators) are easy, that's great! Remember, you still need to practice range of motion to maintain it. As a bonus, while you practice, you also lubricate the shoulder joints with synovial fluid. These "rotators" are also great warm-ups before strenuous upper body activity like lifting weights, shoveling snow, etc.

Range of motion positions are included for the wrists, forearms and fingers as well. That's important because of the negative effects caused by repetitive use of computers, video games and smartphones. Using these devices for countless hours causes the muscles in the forearms, wrists and fingers to progressively tighten (causing muscle imbalance).

The tighter these muscles get, the more likely they are to decrease blood flow and impinge the nerve feeds that supply the hands. That can cause pain, tingling, numbness and restricted blood flow.

Remember, the more time you spend creating a muscle imbalance, the more specific actions you need to take to counteract that detrimental effect. So, if you spend countless hours with technology, you can counteract that effect by practicing the following shoulder and wrist range of motion positions.

Shoulder and Wrist Practice Positions

When we sit hunched over, our shoulders tend to internally rotate (turn toward the middle). Practicing external rotation with the following position is an effective way to counteract this muscle imbalance.

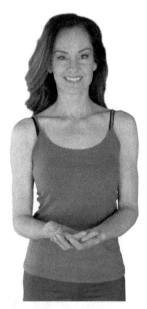

Shoulder Rotator (A)

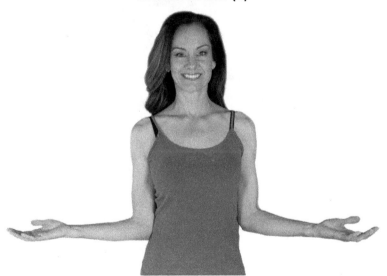

Shoulder Rotator (B)

(A) Tuck the elbows in at the sides. The hands are palms up directly in front of you in line with the belly button. (B) The shoulders externally rotate as the hands move away from the body's center. Alternate between positions (A) and (B).

Shoulder Rotators Continued:
As an experiment, try a few repetitions just on your right side while placing the left hand on top of the right shoulder. This is a good way to check and feel the rotation that is actually happening in the right shoulder joint.

Then go back to rotating both shoulders at one time. If you feel sore or restricted, go less far in either direction until there is no discomfort. Go slowly and accept the range of motion the body allows. You can try up to 20 repetitions. If you want to use soup cans or super light dumbbells, that's fine, but it's not required. By practicing the simple act of rotation, you lubricate the joint with synovial fluid, and maintain range of motion and function.

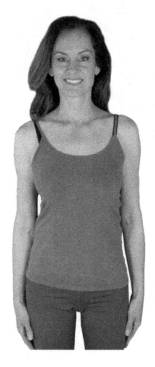

Wings (A)

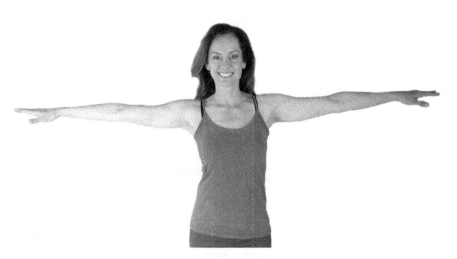

Wings (B)

(A) Stand and let your arms rest at your sides. (B) Then raise your arms up slightly below shoulder height. You alternate between positions (A) and (B). This should not be strenuous. For the recommended number of repetitions, see *Part Four: Let's Practice!*

The idea is to pump blood into your shoulders and one particular rotator cuff muscle (supraspinatus). You activate these muscles because they have leverage to stabilize and protect your shoulder joints.

If Wings feels challenging, then do not do this one every day! You want to give your muscles a chance to recover. If Wings feels easy, then it's okay to do this every day. This is a great warm-up for your shoulders as well before any more strenuous activity.

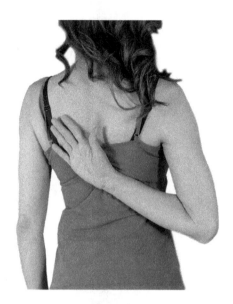

Back Scratch:
Gently guide one hand behind the back to the opposite side until you feel a slight stretch. It can be a struggle to put the hand behind the back at all.

Definitely under-do this stretch for several weeks before increasing it! Give the shoulder time to get used to it. If this position is super easy (which is pretty rare), then you will not need to practice it. You could occasionally check back just to make sure you are maintaining range of motion.

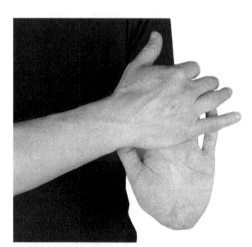

Hand Push Back:
Push the palm of the right hand against the upper part of the palm on the left hand. Slowly push the left hand so that it bends backward until you feel a stretch. Remember to practice both sides.

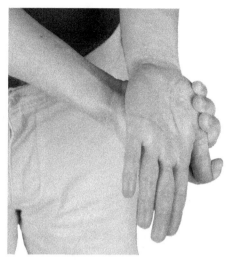

Wrist Rotate (A):
Turn the left palm face up.
The right hand comes underneath
the left. Wrap three fingers
(pinkie, ring, middle) of the
right hand around the thumb
and palm of the left hand.
Slowly rotate the left hand
away from your body.
Remember to practice
both sides.

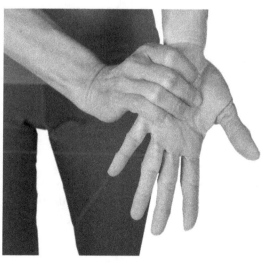

Wrist Rotate (B):
Turn the left palm
face down. Place the
right hand on top of the
left. Wrap four fingers of
the right hand around
the outside of the left
hand. Slowly rotate the left
hand toward your body.

Neck Range of Motion

Picture your skull as a platter full of dishes. When the platter is off-center, it's a lot harder to balance the dishes. When our skull is off-center (usually too far forward), then our upper back and neck muscles tighten to try to stop the head's forward shift.

Normal & Forward Head Position

Head Forward:
The forward head position can restrict blood flow to neck muscles and your brain. This muscle imbalance improves by releasing upper front muscles and activating upper back muscles. Congratulations, you have already learned how to do that!

Perhaps you may have experienced neck issues. For example, you might have difficulty sleeping on a particular side in bed. It may be difficult to look over your shoulder when you back up your car. You may notice stiffness and pain from hours of sitting or tend to get a crick in your neck.

As with all the other joints in this system, the series of interconnected joints in the neck (and supporting muscles) benefit by practicing range of motion. The following neck range of motion positions will help you create better stability, blood flow and function. As a result, that tells the neck it doesn't need to set off the aches and pains alarm.

The neck can be an especially sensitive area. Go easy on it, especially when you first begin to practice. For the recommended stretch time and number of repetitions, see *Part Four: Let's Practice!*

Neck Range of Motion Practice Positions

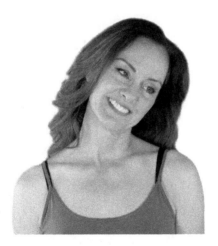

Leaning Neck:
It's useful to practice this position in front of a mirror. Try to keep the chin parallel with the floor. Slowly let one ear move down to the shoulder on the same side. Minimize the stretch, especially when you first begin practicing this position.

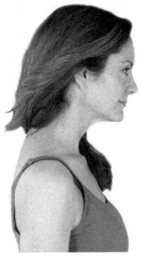

Head Pull Back (A)

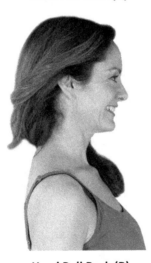

Head Pull Back (B)

A) Stand and allow your head and neck to relax forward. (B) Then move the back of your head backward while keeping the chin parallel to the floor. Pause for a second, then relax and let your head and neck relax forward again (A). You alternate between positions (A) and (B). This position is great for counteracting a head position that is too far forward. Then it's easier to balance that platter full of dishes!

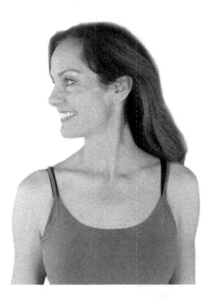

Neck Rotation:
Stand with your chin parallel to the floor. Slowly rotate your head so that your chin moves toward one shoulder. Then slowly rotate the head and chin toward the opposite shoulder. For the recommended number of repetitions, see *Part Four: Let's Practice!*

PART FOUR

LET'S PRACTICE!

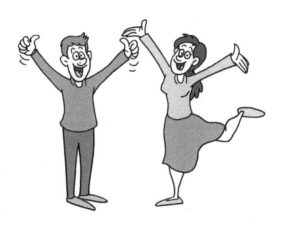

Most clients I work with agree on one main principle: They want fast results. When I first met Sean, I felt exactly the same! Even when it's just aches and soreness, people often want what Sean used to call "a magic bullet" to immediately fix things. Sometimes, people tend to rush or overdo positions to get there faster. That can cause pain and discomfort.

Before buying a product or service, it's common to ask the question, "What's the catch?" So, I will tell you right now. This is not a one-day-and-you're-done proposition. **This system is a quick, daily activity that provides major body benefits for your entire life. However, the long-term plan requires daily practice.**

In particular, the longer you have had a weak point, the more patient and careful you need to be. Your body will tell you how to proceed as long as you are going slowly and easily enough to listen. Could you feel better in some areas quickly, even in one week? Absolutely! But the greatest benefits come from practicing this system for the long term. The goal is not to achieve instant perfection, but to progressively notice improvement and feel better using your body.

By starting off slow and easy, you give yourself time to learn which positions (and corresponding body parts) are weak points. That's useful knowledge. It's much better to know your problem areas before you throw too much at them. By taking your time, you build rapport with your body. That way it becomes less likely to create annoying symptoms like soreness, swelling, aches and pains.

It's helpful to classify the positions in four possible categories:

1) Easy
2) Some room for improvement
3) Weak point (for more information on weak points see page 37)
4) Persistent pain. As you practice, you will become an expert on your parts. You may notice, for example, that your right shoulder is a "1" and your left shoulder is a "3." Your neck could be a "2" and your right hip is a "4."

Never force a position that is a "4" (or any position, for that matter). Pain creates inflammation, more pain and stops improvement. Persistent pain is a message from your body telling you not to do that position! When working with clients, I will never have them do a position that is painful. **If you have any parts that you notice are a "4," your best bet is to hire a health practitioner to help you fix the cause of the problem.**

Also keep in mind that you don't get extra improved function by developing hyper-flexible muscles or excessive joint range of motion. In fact, that can be detrimental to body function.

Individualize Your Practice

As you practice, remember to individualize the positions in categories 1–3. For example, it's fine if you only feel comfortable holding a stretch for five seconds. Or if you notice your right hip is tighter than your left, then don't try to force it to be the same. You can still practice, improve over time and eventually have similar flexibility and joint range of motion on both sides. Remember to practice each position with both sides of your body!

In fact, you may notice that one side of your body is tighter. This is often related to a body part which experienced trauma and/or muscle imbalance from a consistent activity. For example, the upper right side of my body was much tighter than the left. That was caused by injuries to the right side related to a consistent activity (years of right-side-dominated muscles used to play tennis). At the time, I didn't have a plan to counteract all the muscle imbalances I was causing.

Thanks to Sean, I learned how to create muscle balance and effective joint range of motion to improve. You now have learned the same skills to improve function and avoid aches and pains!

Remember this is not a workout! This is your own 28-point inspection: a 10-minute system to target important mechanical parts and take positive actions to benefit them. Benefits include:

- Identify and improve weak points and prevent injuries.
- Create more stable, long-lasting, rock star joints.
- Improve blood flow and shock absorption with improved flexibility.
- Create a healing and more energetic state.
- Tune up body mechanics to feel better, use your body more, and get leaner!

You don't have to suffer, sweat and spend tons of time to get these benefits. You do need to practice consistently! That being said, if you need to take a day off from any of the positions, then that's what you do. For example, your hip muscles may feel stiff when you first start stretching them. Then it's fine to take a day(s) off from the hip stretches.

You also may notice that some of the stretching positions are super easy for you. If so, then you don't need to practice those particular positions. You could just check in periodically to make sure you are maintaining that flexibility.

Practice Light

I highly recommend you **start with "Practice Light" or even less.** You know your body. Just start with what feels comfortable, even if it's just a few of the positions.

"Practice Light" will benefit you as long as you keep practicing. Once you have it down, you can use it as a quick, effective tool: at home, while traveling, before and after playing sports, at the office or the gym. By using "Practice Light," you will be able to tell yourself at the end of each day that you did something to truly benefit your amazing mechanical parts!

Practice Medium and Medium+

You may notice over time that "Practice Light" is easy to run through. Perhaps you even enjoy practicing for longer periods of time or twice a day. That's perfectly fine. More practice leads to more benefits and gives you extra time to improve weak points.

For this reason, Practice Medium and Medium+ are included as an option. They each contain a majority of the exact same positions that are in "Practice Light." However, they both take around 15 minutes and include extra positions for the shoulders, neck, hips and spine. Practice Medium+ is the longer and more challenging option of the three.

Be kind to yourself and adjust your daily practice to how your body feels that day. You may notice your body struggles a little more with the system after being sick, worn down or if you have missed several days of practice.

With each practice plan, the order of the positions is important!

— For example, you warm up the hips with Hip Rotators before practicing hip stretching.

— You warm up the shoulders with Shoulder Rotators before practicing upper front stretching (which can be challenging for the shoulders).

— You warm up the ankles with Toe Circles before practicing quadriceps stretching on the couch (which can be challenging for the ankles).

— You stretch upper front muscles before practicing neck positions. That allows the neck to be in a more balanced position with the upper body before practicing neck stretching and range of motion.

Water and Warm-up

Before you practice please always remember to do the following two things: **1) drink water 2) warm up.**

Our bodies are mostly made up of water. Therefore, all body functions benefit from staying hydrated. This includes **brain function, lubricating joints, elimination, regulating temperature, nutrient absorption, removing toxins and increasing metabolism (the rate at which you burn calories).**

On the other hand, dehydration can cause a wide range of symptoms. These include sluggishness, brain fog and decreased strength and flexibility. Therefore, one of the first questions I routinely ask my clients is, "How much water did you drink today?"

You may have heard that if you don't change your car's oil, it becomes thicker and harder on the engine. The same principle applies with our bodies. When you are dehydrated, your blood becomes thicker, which is harder on your heart and circulatory system. **Always make sure you are hydrated especially before any form of exercise! You wouldn't want to increase demand on a heart which is already struggling because of dehydration!**

It's difficult to say you need to drink exactly "x" amount because that number can vary greatly depending on the individual. For example, a 300-pound professional football player will have a much higher water requirement than a 120-pound office worker who rarely moves. Your body dehydrates the more you eliminate, sweat, drink caffeine and breathe (particularly drier air). Increased weight, activity level and metabolism can also cause you to dehydrate faster.

Tips for Staying Hydrated

A great time to drink water is first thing in the morning since your body dehydrates throughout the night. Try putting a full water bottle by your bed the night before, so in the morning you can rehydrate as quickly as possible.

Always make sure you are hydrated before your workout. It's a lot easier for your heart to push blood through your system when you are hydrated. You will also decrease the potential for injury, and gain power and flexibility.

Coffee, caffeinated tea and soda don't count as water intake. In fact, they dehydrate you faster!

Staying hydrated helps your body detoxify and also delivers nutrients from food and supplements. It even helps deliver caffeine better. If you suspect you are dehydrated, try drinking water with your coffee and you will notice the caffeine works more efficiently to pep you up.

Common initial signs of dehydration can include: a dry mouth and skin, not peeing very much and darker urine (your urine may also be a darker color if you are taking supplements).

Add a twist of lemon, lime, cucumber, or berries to your water. A little flavor makes it easier to drink.

Use a water filter to remove chlorine, which is used to kill living things in the water like bacteria and viruses. Plus, the water will taste better.

Eat fruits and vegetables which have a high water content. You are essentially getting water that has been filtered through a plant, so you get clean water plus vitamins and minerals!

Warm-up

It's ideal to always warm up before running through the Jiffy Body system. If you warm up a piece of taffy, it's easier to bend. It's the same principle with your body. Warmer muscles are more pliable and easier to work with. Proper warm-up is especially beneficial before focusing on any weak points you may have. You could do any light and easy activity for 5 to 7 minutes to get the blood flowing. For example, you could go for a walk.

Build the Habit: Tricks

Improvement is contagious and can motivate you to keep practicing. However, when you feel better, it's also easy to stop. You may decide everything is good now and you can just get on with your life.

I have been guilty of this! Once I had fixed my own body with Sean's help, I decided to play tennis competitively again. I went for a couple of years without any problems and then slacked off of practicing this system regularly. I ended up injuring my back so badly that I had to lie on the floor for three days to allow a pinched nerve to calm down.

Remember the formula for success is
Jiffy Body + Daily Practice = Better Body Function.

As you consistently practice over time, you may notice that some or all of the positions become comfortable and easy to implement. You could practice those types of positions at different points in the day to keep building the habit.

— While you are working in the kitchen, you could do standing positions.

— When a telemarketer calls, that's a good reminder to practice three positions.

— Practice floor positions while watching television, making phone calls or reading a book (dogs, cats, and kids love it when you choose this option). As you become more accustomed to hanging out on the floor, that is a good sign that your body is becoming more functional. Plus, getting up and down from the floor is an important skill and another indicator of your body's mechanical health.

— If it's 10 p.m. and you suddenly realize you forgot to practice the entire day, then do at least one position before bed. **It's so critical to build the habit!**

Once you skip one day, it's too easy to skip more days after that. However, if you do even a little bit every day for 30 days, then you are way more likely to continue. Use this system as a daily part of your life so you can get all of the amazing benefits!

Practice Light

Following is the 10-minute daily system that provides lifetime benefits for muscles and joints. This includes feet, ankles, knees, hips, wrists, shoulders, spine and neck. You improve and maintain body function by 1) practicing joint range of motion and 2) creating and maintaining muscle balance.

The page number next to each position refers to the easiest option for that position and a description of proper form. **It's also a good reminder of the purpose and benefit of practicing.**

Get used to the easiest option of each position first. After you have become accustomed to it over time, **you could eventually pick a more challenging option (particularly for the stretching positions).**

It may take longer to go through Practice Light as you learn it. Once you get it down, you can run through everything in 10 minutes. Practice each position with both sides of the body.

There are recommendations for the length of time to hold a stretch and the number of repetitions for the range of motion positions. Feel free to do less, especially at first. With daily practice, you can easily assess the right amount for you.

It is helpful to use pages 120-123 to quickly practice the system and to avoid overlooking any of the positions.

<u>Standing Positions: Practice Light</u>

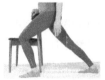

Straight Leg Calf (page 50) (15 seconds)

Bent Leg Calf (page 52) (15 seconds)

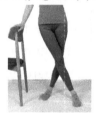

Crossover (page 63) (15 seconds)

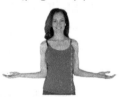

Shoulder Rotator (page 97) (20 repetitions)

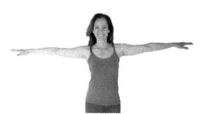

Wings (page 98) (20 repetitions)

Upper Front Stretch (page 86) (15 seconds)

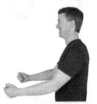

Row Boat (page 93) (20 repetitions)

Reaching Elbow (page 89) (15 seconds)

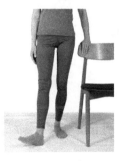

Hip Rotator (page 66) (10 repetitions)

Neck Rotation (page 105) (4 repetitions)

<u>Couch Positions: Practice Light</u>

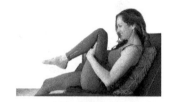

Wishbone (page 74) (15 seconds)

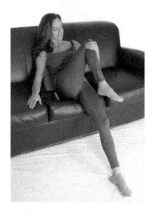

Hip (page 68) (15 seconds)

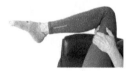

Toe Circles (page 49) (4 repetitions in each direction)

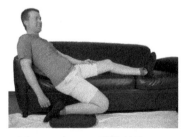

Quadriceps (page 58) (15 seconds)

<u>Floor Positions: Practice Light</u>

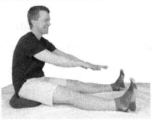

Hamstrings (page 60) (15 seconds)

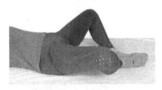

Butterfly (page 62) (15 repetitions to warm up;
15 seconds to stretch)

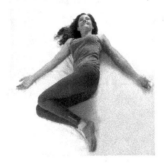

Spine Rotation (page 81) (15 seconds)

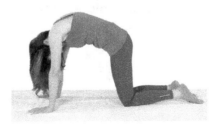

Round and Arch (page 83) (4 repetitions)

Practice Medium

Practice Medium provides the same positions and benefits as Practice Light. It also includes extra positions for the neck, hips, spine and back. A majority of my clients find they enjoy practicing and they obtain further benefit by practicing a few more positions.

Only progress to Practice Medium if Practice Light is easy for you. The page number next to each position refers to the easiest option for that position and a description of proper form. It's also a good reminder of the purpose and benefit for practicing. **By referring back to the book, you also have the option of picking more challenging options, particularly for some of the stretching positions.**

It may take longer to learn Practice Medium at first, but when you get the system down, you can run through everything in around 15 minutes. Practice each position with both sides of the body.

There are recommendations for the length of time to hold a stretch and the number of repetitions for the range of motion positions. Feel free to do less, or more. With daily practice, you can easily assess the right amount for you.

It really is helpful to use pages 125-129 to quickly practice the system and to avoid overlooking any of the positions.

Standing Positions: Practice Medium

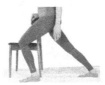

Straight Leg Calf (page 50) (15 seconds)

Bent Leg Calf (page 52) (15 seconds)

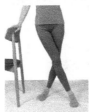

Crossover (page 63) (15 seconds)

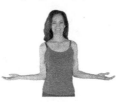

Shoulder Rotator (page 97) (10 repetitions)

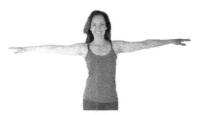

Wings (page 98) (20 repetitions)

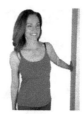

Upper Front Stretch (page 86) (15 seconds)

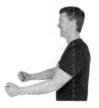

Row Boat (page 93) (20 repetitions)

Reaching Elbow (page 90) (15 seconds)

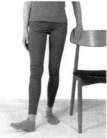

Hip Rotator (page 66) (10 repetitions)

Neck Rotation (page 105) (4 repetitions)

Leaning Neck (page 103) (10 seconds)

Couch Positions: Practice Medium

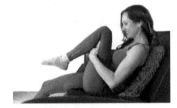

Wishbone (page 74) (15 seconds)

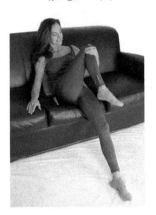

Hip (page 68) (15 seconds)

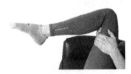

Toe Circles (page 49) (5 repetitions in both directions)

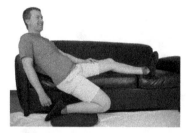

Quadriceps (page 58) (15 seconds)

Chair Position: Practice Medium

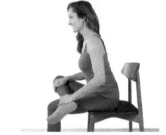

Cross Leg Hip (page 69) (15 seconds)

Floor Positions: Practice Medium

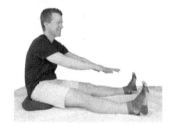

Hamstrings (page 60) (15 seconds)

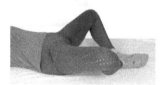

Butterfly (page 62) (20 repetitions to warm up;
20 seconds to stretch)

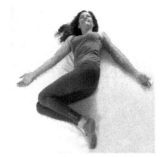

Spine Rotation (page 81) (15 seconds)

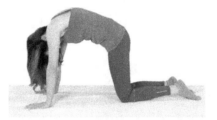

Round and Arch (page 83) (4 repetitions)

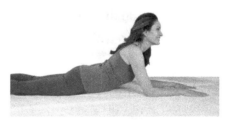

*Spinal Arch (page 80) (15 seconds)

---

* Spinal Arch: If this is super easy, then do not practice this position. That means you already have plenty of lower back arch. You could occasionally check back and try the position to make sure it is still super easy.

Practice Medium+

Practice Medium+ includes extra positions for the shoulders, neck and spine. It is slightly longer and more challenging than Practice Medium.

Only progress to Medium+ if Practice Medium is easy for you. The page number next to each position refers to the easiest option for that position and a description of proper form. It's also a good reminder of the purpose and benefit for practicing. By referring back to the book, **you also have the option of picking more challenging options, particularly for some of the stretching positions.**

It may take longer to learn Practice Medium+ at first, but when you get the system down, you can run through everything in around 15 minutes. Practice each position with both sides of the body.

There are recommendations for the length of time to hold a stretch and the number of repetitions for the range of motion positions. Feel free to do less, or more. With daily practice, you can easily assess the right amount for you.

It really is helpful to use pages 131-136 to quickly practice the system and to avoid overlooking any of the positions.

Standing Positions: Practice Medium+

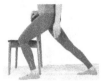

Straight Leg Calf (page 50) (15 seconds)

Bent Leg Calf (page 52) (15 seconds)

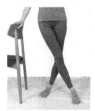

Crossover (page 63) (15 seconds)

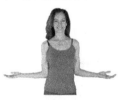

Shoulder Rotator (page 97) (10 repetitions)

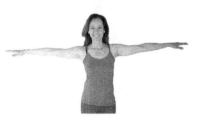

Wings (page 98) (20 repetitions)

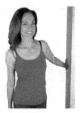

Upper Front Stretch (page 86) (15 seconds)

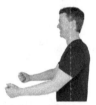

Row Boat (page 93) (20 repetitions)

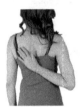

Back Scratch (page 100) (15 seconds)

Reaching Elbow (page 90) (15 seconds)

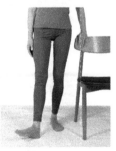

Hip Rotator (page 66) (10 repetitions)

Neck Rotation (page 105) (four repetitions)

Leaning Neck (page 103) (10 seconds)

Head Pull Back (page 104) (4 repetitions)

Couch Positions: Practice Medium+

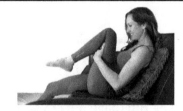

Wishbone (page 74) (15 seconds)

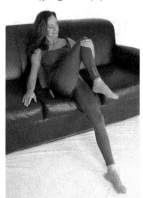

Hip (page 68) (15 seconds)

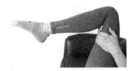

Toe Circles (page 49) (5 repetitions in both directions)

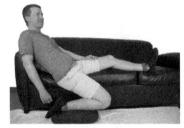

Quadriceps (page 58) (15 seconds)

Chair Position: Practice Medium+

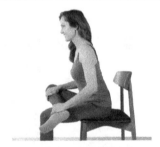

Cross Leg Hip (page 69) (15 seconds)

Floor Positions: Practice Medium+

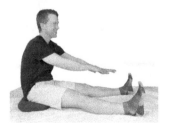

Hamstrings (page 60) (15 seconds)

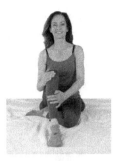

Hip (page 70) (15 seconds)

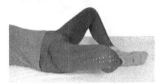

Butterfly (page 62) (20 repetitions to warm up;
20 seconds to stretch)

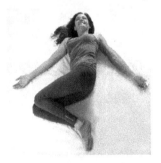

Spine Rotation (page 81) (15 seconds)

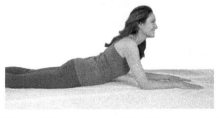

***Spinal Arch** (page 80) (15 seconds)

* Spinal Arch: If this is super easy, then do not practice this position. That means you already have plenty of lower back arch. You could occasionally check back and try the position to make sure it is still super easy.

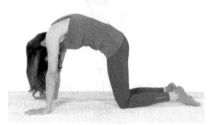

Round and Arch (Spine) (page 83) (4 repetitions)

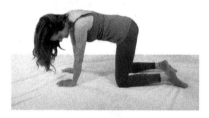

Sideways Spinal (page 82) (15 seconds)

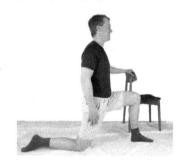

Wishbone (page 76) (15 seconds)

Sitting Break and Better Posture Practice

Counteract muscle imbalance caused by sitting, cell phone and computer use. Create better posture.

The more hours you sit, the more you'll want to use Sitting Break Practice. For example, if you sit five hours a day, you could practice all or some of these positions each time you take a break. As with the other practice plans, adjust how often you practice these positions to accommodate your comfort level.

First, drink water and move around for at least five minutes to improve blood flow. Then use the following positions to:
1. counteract the muscle imbalances caused by excessive sitting and
2. create better muscle balance and posture.

The page number next to each position refers to the easiest option for that position and a description of proper form. It's also a good reminder of the purpose and benefit of practicing.

There are recommendations for the length of time to hold a stretch and the number of repetitions for the range of motion positions. Feel free to do less, especially at first. With daily practice, you can easily assess the right amount for you (and then practice a stretch longer or do more repetitions).

Standing Positions

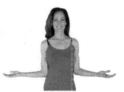

Shoulder Rotator (page 97) (10 repetitions)

Reaching Elbow (page 90) (15 seconds)

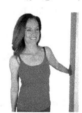

Upper Front Stretch (page 86) (15 seconds)

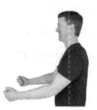

Row Boat (page 93) (10 repetitions)

Hand Push Back (page 100) (15 seconds)
This one is included for counteracting repetitive activities with the hands and wrists, like typing, phone, computer and video games. More wrist range of motion practice positions are also available on page 101.

Couch Position

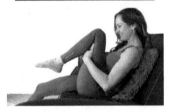

*Wishbone Stretch (page 74) (15 seconds)

Floor Position

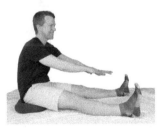

Hamstrings (page 60) (15 seconds)

*The iliopsoas can be stubborn and problematic, so it's always better to ease into stretching it. I recommend you practice the easiest version of this stretch first.

Build the Habit for 30 Days

Make a check for every day you practice for the first 30 days.
You can trick yourself to practice on the days you don't feel like it.
Simply tell yourself you're going to warm up and practice just
three of the positions and then you can stop. Most of the time
you will feel like continuing. But if not, that's okay. You still get
credit!

Your 30-Day Checklist

1	_____	16	_____
2	_____	17	_____
3	_____	18	_____
4	_____	19	_____
5	_____	20	_____
6	_____	21	_____
7	_____	22	_____
8	_____	23	_____
9	_____	24	_____
10	_____	25	_____
11	_____	26	_____
12	_____	27	_____
13	_____	28	_____
14	_____	29	_____
15	_____	30	_____

Identify Your Weak Points

Here is some space to write down the body parts that you need to practice more because they are weak points.

_____

_____

_____

_____

_____

_____

_____

_____

_____

_____

_____

_____

_____

_____

_____

A FINAL THOUGHT:

Do What You Love to Do

A client once told me, "But Bart, I love my yoga class." I responded, "That's great, keep going to yoga!" This system helps you tune up your parts. It also helps you become more knowledgeable about your strengths and weaknesses before enjoying your favorite activities! For example, if you lack shoulder and ankle range of motion, then avoid playing sports until you have tuned up these weak points. Being a weekend warrior is great. Just make sure your living machinery is prepared before slamming on the gas.

Some people even enjoy strength training! They use it to build a more powerful engine resulting in stronger muscles. That creates thicker bones, more stable joints, a sharper mind and they burn body fat in the process.

This 10-minute system is the perfect complement for building a more powerful engine. It helps provide you with better-balanced parts to handle all that power.

Sean used to say the point of spending some time to maintain your body is to help you enjoy life by doing your favorite things. I hope that you will be inspired and ready to start using this system. That way you can experience the lifelong benefits and enjoy staying active with your amazing living machinery!

Acknowledgments

Writing a book is a little bit like climbing a mountain. Just when you think you're getting to the top, you get a better view and realize there's still a "ways" to go. Thanks so much to my family and friends for helping provide that perspective. They gave insightful feedback and encouragement with every draft. To Keziah, thank you for your big picture ideas and endless encouragement. I am grateful to my mother for having always instructed our family with ideas for healthy living and her support of this book all the way through. Thanks to my father and sister for their challenging questions and bright ideas, Hana and Beth for their marketing savvy, and those of you who read this book and provided feedback. Most of all, thank you to my mentor Sean McCarver, the ultimate human body mechanic, who helped me and countless others with his intelligence and dedication.

Visit jiffybody.com/contact to subscribe for a monthly, quick body tip sent straight to your inbox. Get reminders and fresh information to help you keep practicing and improving!

Contact me at bart@jiffybody.com and I will e-mail you this free "cheat sheet" for the Practice Light system and also one for Sitting Break and Better Posture Practice. Clients and readers have requested both handouts so they can post them on their wall. That way they can save time, not skip any positions and feel better faster.

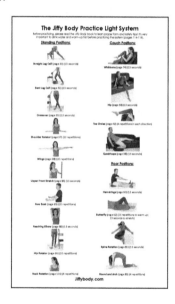